COMMON SENSE

MEDICINE

Published by Lisa Hagan Books 2024

www.lisahaganbooks.com

ISBN: 978-1-945962-63-9

Interior layout by Simon Hartshorne

COMMON SENSE
MEDICINE
MAKING AMERICA HEALTHY AGAIN

DR. LON JONES, DO

Contents

Preface

Before going into medicine, my undergraduate studies in history acquainted me with a big inspiration for the American Revolution, Thomas Paine's incendiary pamphlet *Common Sense.* It fired up the American colonists to revolt against British rule in 1776, making them see the possibility of creating a new nation based on revolutionary ideas. The colonists dared to think of themselves as free people with the God-given right of self-determination, not as British subjects but as Americans. *Common Sense* incited them to direct their *counterwill*—their resistance against unfair, top-down coercion—at King George and his treatment of them as *other*, as less worthy. If not for Paine, the American Revolution may not have happened when it did, or at all.

Taking Paine's ideas and spirit with me during the following decades as a practicing physician, I developed my own brand of revolutionary thinking known as Common Sense Medicine®. It's based on three emerging, yet old, elements (portrayed on this book's cover) that will change the nature of medicine. The first element comes from Hippocrates, the father of Western medicine, who told us that our food should be our medicine. The second element comes from Claude Bernard, the father of modern physiology, who enlightened us to the fact that our natural defenses are just as important as our microbes as a determining factor in the development of illness and disease. The third element comes from Charles Darwin, the father of evolution, who explained for us the processes of natural selection. I apply natural selection to physiology by recognizing that the body's natural defenses are gifts from nature, and rather than suppress them as is common in medical practice today, we should follow Hippocrates by aiding and enhancing them with the right foods.

We can learn a revolutionary way of treating infectious diseases from these forefathers if only we'd stop handicapping our natural defenses with environmental changes and wrongheaded measures. The wrong turn in medical practice happened during the debate between Claude Bernard and Louis Pasteur about the cause of disease. Pasteur argued for the microbe and Bernard argued for the "soil," the place where the microbe is planted, i.e., our bodies. Both of these eminent scientists were right, but Pasteur's argument about supposedly deadly microbes led us to embark on a foolhardy medical war against them that we are still waging today, at the expense of crippling the natural defenses against disease we have all obtained through natural selection. Because of Pasteur's offensive approach, we war against microbes by using pharmaceutical drugs that kill them, instead of taking the defensive approach advocated by Bernard and Hippocrates that would make them commensal—in short, make them our friendly neighbors and allies.

Killing microbes activates their defenses, and it's those defenses that can be so detrimental to humans. Microbial colonies defend themselves by building a safe house inside the body, known as a biofilm. Then they mutate to cope with the threat, and this is when things can get really bad for the human dealing with an infection. The ability of microbes to defend and mutate in response to threat is the source of antimicrobial resistance that's bedeviling medical science today. But creating ever-more powerful antibiotics would be mostly unnecessary if we would learn how to better co-exist with microbes.

We need to better understand our "enemy," and today we can do that because we have better information than Pasteur had. Living within each of us are something in the order of three trillion microbes. We call it the human biome, a community similar to the ecological biomes that support life on Earth, and we treat the human one as badly as we do the ecological ones. Microbes digest our food, protect our bodily openings from outside pathogens, and even aid in our evolutionary development, yet we treat them as enemies. The warfare mentality begun by Pasteur and embraced by profit-driven medical practice now extends to inside our bodies. We are at war with ourselves, and it's a war we cannot win.

Microbes play a profound role in supporting life on this planet. For two billion years, they were the only life here. Then, because the methane environment of the early Earth was an evolutionary dead-end, new microbes developed—cyanobacteria—that harnessed the power of the sun to split the water molecule and make oxygen. Life flourished. The methane-centered microbes went underground where they found safety and produced the natural gas that heats our homes and cooks our food.

Since Pasteur's era, we have also learned how these microscopic organisms not only make life possible but also survive through cooperation, communication, and mutual benefit. Humans, on the other hand, are mutually destroying each other because we don't cooperate or effectively communicate. But microbes have much to teach us that can solve a litany of problems faced by humanity, in particular by studying how they communicate. Microbes, and indeed all microscopic life (with few exceptions) are covered in glycans, long chains of sugars and sugar complexes that coat both plant and animal cells. They are ubiquitous and provide a means of communication in the microscopic world. They tell our developing cells where to go and tell our immune system what is native to the body and what is not. Plus, they trigger a variety of helpful responses in particular situations. The basic cause of many diseases is the body can no longer tell what is native, and it ends up attacking itself.

Glycans were only identified with electron microscopy and specific stains that don't disrupt them, so most of us are only just finding out about them. The science of glycobiology is leading us to better understanding of how infection begins and how we can stop it. But at present, the bureaucratic division between foods and drugs is blocking progress in our use of glycan mimes in our defensive negotiation with microbes.

Glycans are crucial for understanding infection because they are the "docking station" between microbes and human cells, a process known as adherence. Once a microbe adheres to a cell, it begins the process of infection. I discovered how to disrupt that process at the body's openings through the use of xylitol, a natural sugar alternative known in Finland as birch sugar, in a nasal spray. It was a happy accident—at the time, while trying to treat chronic ear infections in babies, I discovered that administering the spray at every diaper change prevented almost all ear infections.

Later, I discovered that it prevents asthma and allergies, too.

This simple way of using food as medicine should be known far and wide, but since xylitol is a food and not an approved drug, no drug claims can be made about it. According to the FDA, foods cannot be called drugs without first going through an expensive approval process. To succeed, the researchers have to tie the working glycan to a patentable, controllable, and therefore profitable protein, in order to pay for FDA approval and open the door to making big profits, so I doubt that anyone will be told which glycan is the key. In the future, scientists are likely be able to use glycans to differentiate between what is us, native to the body, and what is cancer and create a new class of drugs to treat the disease. Pasteur gave us the belief that microbes are a great threat to our health, but the demand for profits is the far greater threat not only to our health but also to our healthcare system.

The paradigm of profit-seeking as the driving force behind medical innovation is seen by many progressive thinkers as likely to morph into a more favorable information-based system, predicated on the sharing of scientific advancements, rather than hoarding them for profit, and at Common Sense Medicine® we are thrilled to be a part of that movement.[1] But for now, we are stuck with a profit-driven system that ignores what Hippocrates taught us, and discourages research.

A significant part of my study's results involves a food, xylitol, that's generally recognized as safe by the FDA. It's the main ingredient in Xlear® (pronounced "clear"), the nasal spray I developed to optimize the body's airway defenses and block many microbes from adhering, including the SARS virus that causes COVID infection. Unfortunately, though, the FDA says that only a drug, not a food, can make such a medical claim. Xylitol is inexpensive and available without a prescription, making it a threat to the drugs on the market which cost much more because they must pass expensive FDA-mandated studies that only pharmaceutical companies can afford. That's the reason you are probably just hearing about it here.

We call foods like xylitol *Hippocratic drugs*, named after Hippocrates. That physician of ancient Greece, whose Oath is still what graduating physicians swear to today, told us that our food should be our drugs. But the use of food as a drug was *de facto* ruled out in 1962 when Congress passed new rules for

FDA-approved drugs to be effective as well as safe. It's *de facto* because showing efficacy requires very expensive clinical, pricing foods out of the FDA 'drug' marketplace. And without FDA approval, the producers and distributors of Hippocratic drugs cannot make any drug claims, so the public remains ignorant of their benefits, and little research is done.

The processes of evolution also play a profound role in all of this. Evolution is how our defenses formed to protect our vulnerable bodily openings from outside attack by microbes. It's also how sugars and their complexes found a niche in enabling our cells and microbes to communicate. But evolution is seen as a threat, a threat not to the drug industry but to religion. Lots of people in America are afraid of evolution for religious reasons, but I don't see it that way. According to James (1:27, KJV): "Pure and undefiled religion before God and the Father is this: to visit orphans and widows in their trouble, and to keep oneself unspotted from the world." Micah asked what God wanted from mankind, and was told "to do justly, and to love mercy, and to walk humbly with your God." Religious people feel threatened by evolution based on ancient, culturally derived explanations for why things are the way they are, explanations that were seen by the wise people of the time as the best available.

But at the core of Common Sense Medicine is a proposal to re-establish the definition of religion handed down to us by James and Micah. We are promoting a paradigm shift that combines power, something well-understood by evolution, with the sort of love that religious people understand and cherish. When Reverend Martin Luther King said, "Power at its best is love implementing the demands of justice, and justice at its best is power correcting everything that stands against love," he spoke of coupling power with love.

Those with power need more love, and in the name of love we need to acquire the power to change what's making America unhealthy.

Along with everyone else, religious people need to see evolution not as a threat, but as the theory that explains the way things change. Charles Darwin observed biological changes that occurred over the span of thousands of years in the bird and other animal specimens he studied, and he summed up his observations in what he called *natural selection*, consisting of three elements: change (mutation), fitness consequences (environmental elements constraining the mutation's success), and reproduction. We know the power behind these three elements. We breed faster horses, change wolves into countless breeds of dogs, and make hybrid crops that are more sustainable, all by controlled breeding. And now that we have CRISPR we can address the mutation process itself. That in-between step, and its application to social change, is largely what this book is about. We can frame the fitness landscape in a variety of ways. Currently in healthcare, profit is the frame, but if we choose to we can substitute well-being Doing so is how we make America healthy again, by using conscious evolution.

Social change follows the same set of rules—rules that can be used to guide society's evolutionary success. Many of our actions as a society are an evolutionary failure, but with more information we can make better choices and fulfill the promise that lit America's revolutionary fire for life, liberty, and the pursuit of happiness.

We can make America healthy again through a commonsense approach that I hope will be as successful as Thomas Paine's revolution. Truly, as he said in his pamphlet that rocked the world, "We have it in our power to begin the world over again."

But the radical changes we so desperately need won't come

from within the system—the powers-that-be like things the way they are because it's making them rich. Change today must come from the people, as it did in 1776. Just as colonial Americans shared Paine's revolutionary pamphlet with each other, you can share the ideas in this book. Knowledge is power when put to good use.

My time on this earth began before the Second World War, and in my long and fruitful life I have played the role of father to 16 children and doctor to many thousands. Now retired from medicine, I have grandchildren and great-grandchildren, and like many people in the autumn of life I am thinking about what I can leave behind to make the world a better place. This is my offering.

Introduction

Around the turn of the 21st century, I began using xylitol mixed in a saline nasal spray. My hope was it would stop my granddaughter's recurring ear infections. It did. I did it because a group of Finnish researchers had showed that chewing xylitol sweetened gum five times a day prevented about half of chronic ear infections, and it did this by preventing the adherence of the microbes.

Encouraged, I ran a study on children experiencing the same problem. Their reports of ear complaints fell by 95% during the year I watched them. I tested xylitol's effectiveness against respiratory infections, and against allergies and asthma. Patients got better.

I was onto something, and it was something different. Asthma and allergies have nothing to do with microbial adherence. I would soon find out why.

I'd found an alternative to the often costly and side-effect-ridden mainstream treatments for a variety of conditions, and I could heal my patients at a fraction of the cost by using a saline spray containing the magic ingredient, xylitol. I knew I was onto a revolutionary treatment for upper respiratory problems, one of the major conditions for which people seek medical care.

Then, the hospital where I practiced medicine closed, and so did my clinic, making it impossible to run more studies, so I turned to the people in government who are supposed to be the experts, the FDA. I called and managed to get a live person on the phone. "I have a very simple and neat way to clean the nose," I said.

The baffled FDA bureaucrat replied, "We don't have a category for nose cleaning. What good does it do?"

My answer was simple. "If your nose is clean, you don't get

infections in your ears or sinuses, and allergies and asthma basically go away."

"Then it's a drug," said the bureaucrat.

And that's when the door to further progress slammed shut. To satisfy the FDA, the price tag for a drug study starts at around a million dollars, and I'd have to finance it myself—and that was only the first hurdle on the road to approval. Even though xylitol mixed with saline is technically a food, the FDA calls it a drug. In *Commonsense Medicine: Healing from the Inside Out and Stopping the Next Pandemic*, the prequel to this book, I spell out why it's a bad idea to put food and drug safety under one roof at the FDA but suffice to say that my case is a prime example. I'd need deep pockets to fund a study for my "food" so that I could call it a drug.

Next, I called on the industry with a monopoly on drugs and plenty of money to fund studies, the pharmaceutical industry. They were intrigued when I told them about my clinical findings, but their interest evaporated the moment they found out that xylitol is the main ingredient. Xylitol is a natural product that cannot be patented, and without a patent, a company cannot claim exclusive rights to make a drug. Those rights allow the drug company to charge enough to recoup the expense of jumping through FDA hoops. No exclusive rights means "sorry, not interested."

Hear the sound of the door slamming? It would have been the end of the story, but people needed to know about my discovery, and I needed a product people could use and tell others about. That's how Xlear® nasal spray was born. FDA-approved drugs are expensive because of the studies demanded to show both safety and efficacy. To pay for them, drug companies pass on the costs to consumers, and if Xlear were to be classified as a drug it would mean jacking up the price to something like $50 per bottle. A prudent patient or business competitor could put a dime's worth of xylitol in a bottle of saline nasal spray and thereby deny the drug company its profits, and everyone in the pharmaceutical industry knows this. Back then, I knew *what* xylitol did, and that it was safe, but not *how* it worked.

Now I know how, and it is revolutionary. It has to do with the body's natural defenses in the airway and how microbes gain a foothold there. The science is clear but ignored by Western medicine, so please, when you read in the coming pages why it is revolutionary, tell your family and friends. As comedian Chris Rock once said when talking about HIV, "There is no money in a cure. The money's in the comeback." Keep 'em coming back for more, back to the pharmacy and its astonishingly high prices. That's why drugs are not designed to cure, they're designed to treat symptoms and keep people coming back. It's why our collective health continues declining despite our marvelous advances in medical science. Keeping your airway defenses at peak efficacy means four sprays a day in each nostril, so a bottle of Xlear should last about four months. A few dollars per month at most to protect the airway from infection and allergens.

But you won't hear about it on the evening news, which means it's up to us—you, me, and the public—to tell our stories and share them with our families, friends, and communities. As it did in 1776, change must come from the people. It's up to us to make America healthy again, starting now.

CHAPTER 1

Our Life-Threatening Emergency

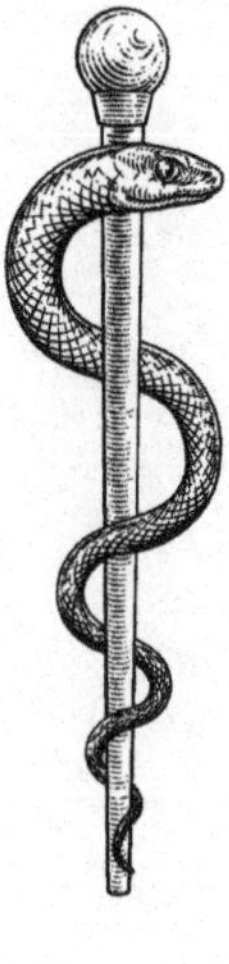

As a doctor, I help people with their health, and a half-century of practicing medicine taught me that health is about much more than addressing symptoms and prescribing treatments. Health is about well-being. Well-being includes not just our physical and emotional condition, but also the security gained through the ability to provide for basic needs. Well-being begins in our environment: our homes, families, communities, and nation. When they are healthy, we are healthy.

Something else I learned as a physician is that microbes respond as a community when they have a problem, but people are largely expected to respond individually, especially in the Western world. If you possess the resources to survive, good for you; otherwise, it's not so good for you. The concept behind universal healthcare rests on the idea of the individual as the agent; it's the agent that needs the help, and it's expensive. But in most cases the environment is the problem, and it needs help if we are to make America healthy again.

All members of a community share the same environment, and the weak and vulnerable are the first to show symptoms when something's wrong. They are the canaries in the coal mine, and they are succumbing. Physically, mentally, and spiritually, entire segments of the population are sick and infected by the toxins in their environment—not just chemical toxins but also social, economic, political, and environmental. They impact our well-being. After an infection takes hold, it attacks healthy parts of the body. The health of the collective body, the body politic, is under attack, too, and we are past the tipping point.

The decline in well-being is seen most dramatically in life expectancy, an established standard for measuring the quality of a healthcare system. After many decades of increases in US life expectancy, it essentially went flat around 2010, and started declining in 2019. In medicine, a patient is admitted to intensive care when their health takes such a serious turn in the wrong direction, but intensive care will only save us if we expand our focus beyond the individual to include the complex interrelationship between ourselves and our environment. There is no simple drug, medicine, or food that will fix this patient's health woes. Restoring our collective health requires paradigm changes in culture and society, and that comes from simple and beneficial information understood and acted on by all. Government can help if we change its focus from improving the GDP to improving society's health, but the incentive and initiative for that change must come from the people. At present, our government is just as sick as we are, taken over from within by a parasitic infection with a dollar sign.

In its quest to survive, a parasite infects the host and finds ways to complete its life cycle, and in some cases, things turn out all right. But in other cases, the results are fatal for the host organism. Our nation is like an organism, with social parasites—the agents that use society for their own benefit, with no regard for collective health—that go through their life cycle at its expense. Some social parasites are like single-cell protozoa that live in the gut and don't cause problems, resulting in a 'live and let live' homeostasis, but others cause sickness. American society is sick and suffering from a parasitic infection, and it won't get better until the parasite is removed—or tamed.

Social parasites infect us with their beliefs and ideas, like might makes right, the law of the jungle, and survival of the fittest. Living in an environment where these are the rules of the game pushes us into a state of heterostasis, an imbalance where the body can no longer hold off the infection. When the tipping point is reached the infection takes over. We become like the mice infected with *Toxoplasma*, a common parasite that doesn't seem to bother humans, but in mice it gets into their brains and removes their fear. They don't run from cats anymore. Those of us infected by social parasites lose our ability to discern threats to our well-being.

Virulence is the medical term for when microbes become dangerous to us, and it's always related to how easily they can spread. It's true for social infections, too, so we must stop the spread, and it begins with how we think and what we believe.

Social parasites infect our thinking, but they also force us to serve their interests. In nature, a parasite works from within the host organism to make it act in ways that favor the parasite and wreak destruction on the host. Our society is the host for social parasites controlling us from within. The infection is in the body politic. Our social parasites know exactly where to target to continue spreading: our government and other social institutions. We need only consider the fact that for every elected official in Washington, DC, there are 24 lobbyists—24 to 1. In 2022, those lobbyists spent $4 billion peddling their influence.[2] Infected by the parasite, our elected officials are like mice that stop acting in the public interest, even to the point of death-by-cat. They no longer serve the interests of the people who elect them, and instead they become slaves to the financial interests that infect them with their beliefs and greed. As mouthpieces for their industry sponsors, they influence the very ways that we, on the receiving end of their propaganda, think. This is why nothing less than changing the paradigm will save us.

As a result of this infection, our societal structures and systems are in terrible trouble, so much so that it threatens our nation's existence as a democratic republic. If we are to save ourselves, we need our government to reevaluate its purpose: to form a more perfect union (not happening), establish justice (for those who can afford it), ensure domestic tranquility (at the expense of the highest rate of incarceration in the developed world), provide for the common defense (by focusing only on an expensive offense), promote the general welfare (look at our poverty rate), and secure the blessings of liberty to ourselves and our posterity (as long as one is in the dominant caste).

We really can do better by applying the fitness characteristics, that constrain what works in evolution, to our public policies, so that they work in our favor rather than for the social parasites. Doing that is what we call "conscious evolution." It's the conscious application of what evolution can teach us about society.

Which raises the question, why isn't it happening already? And the answer is that the quest for economic power through the accumulation of wealth outweighs the importance of the nation's health, resulting in sickness.

My brand of commonsense medicine promotes personal health alongside societal health, and both are close to their death beds. Our defenses against the social parasites are worn down, and so too are the physiological defenses that sustain our personal health. Ignored for too long, the bill has come due, but it's manageable when we have the right understanding.

This is our life-threatening emergency, and unlike the voices telling us only how dire the situation is, in this book we will hear from voices offering solutions that piggyback atop the understanding gained from evolution and the revolutionary scientific understanding of how microbes, the original life on this planet, survive. Telling us how bad things are without offering solutions is intentionally designed to put us under stress, clouding our thinking and making us reactive instead of careful and deliberative. It benefits the parasite, which can then speak through the mouths of our leaders and other influencers to push us in the direction of serving its interests, not ours, and we go along with it because we are infected, too.

FROM DIAGNOSIS TO CURE

This book is about our nation's health and the ways we can promote it. Claude Bernard, the father of modern physiology, and Hippocrates, the father of Western medicine, taught us that individual health is a collective issue. It's holistic, more than just symptoms treated tactically with band-aid solutions, and so is our nation's health. And the principles and strategies of defense medicine can cure it, just as they do for our personal health.

Later, we will discuss the ill thinking of Social Darwinism, the problems caused by capitalism, and the short-sighted decision-making driven by the stress response, but first we must understand why we are vulnerable in the first place. Like the human body, the body politic can stand up against invaders when its defenses are optimized, but currently they are not. In short, we are vulnerable because, as we have done with our physiological defenses, we have likewise ignored our social defenses.

The correlation is strong between the "whys" for the crippling of both our personal and social defenses, and it comes down to the corrupting influence of money and the financial benefits of gaming the system. Our healthcare system benefits financially from illness and the warfare mentality against microbes. Powerful elements of our society benefit from the flocking response of the public to the perception of threat, so they create more threats, crisis after crisis, some real and some imagined, to keep us in fight mode and thus vulnerable. As our leaders often say: don't let a crisis go to waste. Crisis creates vulnerabilities that can be exploited, which social parasites see as opportunities.

The Chinese character for crisis is made from combining the characters for "danger" and "change point." It's appropriate as a symbol for the chaos we face today. The danger we all sense is making us focus on fighting the opposition and spending outrageous amounts of money doing so. Elements in society positioned to take advantage of the changes profit immensely, incentivizing them to continue hammering away at society's weakened defenses. But crisis is also a trigger for ideas and mutations where solutions may emerge—for changes in response to the danger.

The crisis we are in presents an opportunity for the changes we need to make as a nation, but the response to the emergence of COVID-19 epitomizes the ugly side of this dynamic. First, we were presented with the danger of the virus, but were told it was just like the flu. Fear of it spread rapidly. The healthcare and drug industries tooled up to fight it, but to make that goose lay its golden eggs required them to take less expensive alternatives off the table. Evidence from sufficient studies supported the possibility that ivermectin and hydroxychloroquine—inexpensive generic drugs—worked against the virus, but they were not FDA-approved for that purpose, and that became the wedge driven into the public's mind to scare them away. Giants in the healthcare industry, positioned to take advantage of the pandemic with their much more costly solutions, argued loudly against the alternatives because their own solutions could only be approved as they emerged, and that category required the absence of alternatives. And they enjoyed the support of those they financially sponsor, not only in the regulatory agencies of government, but also the mainstream media, which gladly hyped the fear to maximum effect.

Early on during the pandemic, a puzzling fact emerged from Africa. Across the continent, relatively few people were getting sick from COVID, but they were getting infected. Tests showed the presence of COVID antibodies across the population. They must have had a natural resistance to the virus, and evolutionary history tells us why. Our airways adapted to the humid, tropical environments present across swaths of the African continent, where humanity "grew up" before migrating, and are still tuned to work in optimally humid environments, enabling airway defenses to do their job against viruses and other invaders. Those natural defenses are the combination of the mucins, that hold on to all pollutants, and the cilia—microscopic hairs—that sweep it out. Both are dependent on the airway surface fluid, which comes from the water in the air we breathe when the ambient humidity is greater than 40% RH, which is normal in the forested areas of Africa. And the mucins also contain the same glycans as those the microbes are looking to attach to on our cell surfaces.

In Africa and many other places where our defenses are working optimally the virus enters the nose as we breathe, finds what it is looking for in the mucin glycans, sticks to them, is passed by immune cells on the way to the stomach, and then also triggers more immunity in the GI tract on the way out. Immunity and antibodies are developed without ever making the person sick. Which is how it should work.[3] But in places where air conditioning is in widespread use, water is removed from the indoor air, making us more vulnerable to airborne infection. Air conditioning is not widespread in Africa but is in other parts of the world where the virus rampaged through the population.

Another factor that gave Africans an advantage against the virus is the widespread use of ivermectin to treat and prevent river blindness. When news first leaked that ivermectin was effective against COVID, systemic resistance against it cranked into action by calling it horse medicine, but it's certainly not just a horse medicine as our ill-informed media would have us believe. Ivermectin is an old, safe, and inexpensive drug. It's used to deworm animals and prevent river blindness. When farmers and vets started using it for COVID, the FDA ignored its safe use in humans and published the warning about using animal drugs, completely ignoring the data emerging from Africa showing that the regions with endemic river blindness, where ivermectin was in wide use, had minimal cases of COVID. But the FDA required their standard double-blind, placebo-controlled studies to show efficacy, and—surprise, surprise—ivermectin's patent had expired, so anyone could make it, no one could control it financially, and with a profit motive, no one stepped up to pay for the demanded tests.

But even if the argument is correct that ivermectin was not as effective in treating COVID as initially thought, the fact that its use was downplayed from the get-go once again speaks volumes. The world was in crisis and the vaccines were still in testing, but we had shelves full of safe medicine, backed by evidence of efficacy, ready to deploy. Would it have hurt to at least try? But "Operation Warp Speed" was in effect, and its 'emergency use authorization' would not pass muster if there were alternative treatments. By the time the *New England Journal of Medicine* weighed in with a study concluding that the efficacy of ivermectin in the treatment of COVID was "inconsistent," we were already well into 2022, but the authors acknowledged the strong supporting evidence for efficacy from other studies. Plus, they only studied high-risk patients.[4] Perhaps ivermectin wouldn't have been effective against COVID in high-risk cases, but evidence suggests otherwise when used to treat infected people whose health is relatively good.

President Trump was justly criticized after suggesting the use of disinfectants to prevent SARS-COV-2 infection, but he would have hit the mark by instead saying preservatives. Lab tests have shown that a variety of preservatives such as grapefruit-seed extract, which is also used as a disinfectant, have strong antiviral and antimicrobial effects and disable the SARS virus. But they are Hippocratic drugs—foods with drug effects—that Big Pharma won't back. That industry's self-interested, profit-demanding way of thinking scoffs at the use of these agents, and as a result countless lives are lost. It's a prime example of bureaucratic culture, one where "emphasis is on the policies, rules, and compliance," and where Hippocratic drugs are either unwelcome or ignored.[5]

(It's also interesting to note that ivermectin and grapefruit-seed extract kill parasites, and it makes us wonder if the parasite that's infected the minds of decision-makers influenced them, because logically it makes no sense to not even try these alternatives during an epic crisis. Remember, a parasite controls from within, changing the way the host organism thinks and behaves.)

Our bureaucratic culture will continue blocking the cures we need. Self-interested industries whose profit margins are threatened by alternatives will continue blocking them. Even in the face of our life-threatening emergency, the status quo keeps its grip, compelling us to ask how much worse things must get before enough of us demand change. In science, there's an old adage that change happens one funeral at a time, meaning that the old guard must die off before new ideas and ways of thinking have any chance of gaining acceptance. The old guard built their reputations and careers around consensus opinions and practices. It's true not only in science but also across societal institutions, and the reasons for it boil down to the quest for power, and the single-minded pursuit of self-interest.

We can't wait for the old guard to pass the torch. Our way of doing things is making us sick, and it's worsening. To make America healthy again, we will start by taking a fresh look at an old idea: evolution.

CHAPTER 2

Beginning Again with Evolution

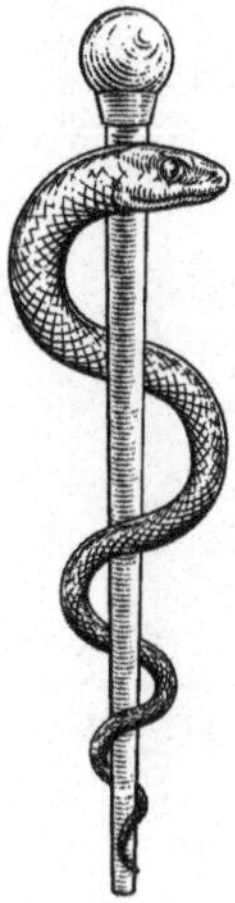

Most of us are aware of natural selection. Beneficial mutations that enhance survival benefits spread throughout the population via reproduction. That's what evolution is all about, but it's too revolutionary for some, like the fellow traveler I once spoke with. He thought it reasonable as I explained how natural selection works, until I said "evolution." Evolution ran counter to his religious beliefs, shutting down the discussion.

But evolution is a fact, and it's just as applicable to nations and societies as it is to biology. Evolution has three elements: change (both genetic and memetic); fitness characteristics (the environment that constrains the change's success); and reproduction (the ability to spread). All three elements can be played with to benefit biology and society. We can come up with new ideas, both good and bad, but fitness characteristics are the elements in the environment that the change must satisfy to be successful. Biologically, reproduction can be blocked—such as by using a condom to prevent the spread of STDs—and culturally we can prevent the spread of infectious ideas and beliefs in the body politic. Evolution is our map to follow to make America healthy again.

The idea behind playing with fitness characteristics comes from the work of Paul Ewald and his book *Evolution of Infectious Disease*. When he showed that the path for the spread of mutating microbes is either through virulence (when transmission is easy) or commensalism (when it is not), he not only described their fitness landscape but also how it can be played with for our benefit. Any means that impedes transmission pushes the organism to live with its current host in a friendlier, win-win way. That's what commensalism means—living better with each other, and it applies to society as well as to microbes. Our defenses against social parasites begin with blocking transmission of their beliefs and ways of thinking and behaving.

There are many similarities between the mutations that begin the changes in nature and the ideas that do the same in society. The similarities are not in the nature of the changes but in the processes leading to their success, though there is a big caveat: Nature's fitness landscape is selected based on what aids survival, and the benefit is gained by both the individual and also the group or species, but in society the landscape is shaped artificially based on what increases personal profits or gives a power advantage. One's profit solely for self-interest or political advantage may benefit a small cohesive group where a powerful leader has credibility, but it's a loss for the larger and more diverse communities that make up our country, and it goes against nature. The principles of evolution are just as easy to abuse as they are to apply for our benefit.

Fitness characteristics passed on through genetics are what help organisms and their groups increase survival and reproduction. Memetic evolution is that of ideas, and their survival and spread are determined by an open marketplace, assuming it exists in the first place. The marketplace is our best parallel for the fitness landscape of nature, but unlike nature it is easily manipulated. One glaring example is the preference for expensive COVID treatments over less expensive alternatives. It's not what an open marketplace would choose; it was the choice of the people looking to make huge profits. The influence of big money can change society's fitness landscape to further augment the profits and power of the wealthy, so let's look into the relationship between money and power.

THE COLLUSION OF POWER

Power is the game we're playing in our society, and the quest for it is the basis of our civilization. J.K. Rowling's character Voldemort summed it up well when he said, "There is no good and evil, there is only power, and those too weak to seek it." We all know who Voldemort (Harry Potter's nemesis) is, and there are many who resist seeking power because of its association with evil. Law professor Sherrilyn Ifill said in the New York Review of Books:[6]

> Progressive people often seem averse to the pursuit of power. It is as though we think "power" is a bad word. We think it unseemly. We worry, perhaps appropriately, about how power can corrupt and harm. But that is what happens when people abuse their power. It is not power's natural tendency. We must believe enough in our own integrity to trust ourselves with power. "Power without love is reckless and abusive," Dr. Martin Luther King Jr. famously said, "and love without power is sentimental and anemic. Power at its best is love implementing the demands of justice, and justice at its best is love correcting everything that stands against love."

Our goal should be the beneficial use of power, and in later chapters we will find ways to accomplish that, but first the historian in me wants to know how we got here. What mistakes do we need to learn from, and when did *power* become a problem?

Despite our misbelief that we are separate from nature, we are not; and we can learn much from nature. There is no power problem in nature, there are only niches where organisms find their means of survival. There are alpha species at the top of their food chains, but they don't store up their food to gain more power like humans do, and that's where humans made the mistake of breaking away from nature and its example, and power started becoming a problem.

Early human societies were egalitarian, according to *Survival of the Friendliest*, a book by Brian Hare and Vanessa Woods. They look at what we know about early hominid societies going back to nearly one hundred thousand years ago, when *Homo erectus* seemed the most fit. This ancestor of modern humans was strong and knew how to use fire and make stone tools, and its heritage stretched back a million years. But over the next twenty-five thousand years they lost out to the *Neanderthals*, who were more social. Then they were overcome by the *Homo sapiens,* who had developed better technology in both weapons (knives, barbed hooks, and spears) and domestication (ovens and food storage). They also formed larger groups and were less mobile, but Hare and Wood argue that the deciding difference was what they called "cooperative communication." *Homo sapiens* "were able to self-domesticate in the healthy pathway."[7] Until recently, we also assumed that defeats in battle led to the demise of Neanderthals, but we're finding out from ancient DNA that the changes were evolutionary and caused more by mixed sexual relations than by violence.

Carrying that forward to early human communities, we find that the earliest civilizations were built around cooperation. In *The Dawn of Everything*, anthropologist David Graeber and archaeologist David Wengrow argue that contrary to popular understanding, early cities were not divided into social classes and hierarchies. These communities grew through the cooperative communication proposed by Hare and Woods. Not only does the archaeological evidence support their case, but simple logic does, too. The people living in early civilizations had nowhere else to go. When living together is not just the best but really the only option, people learn to cooperate. Similarly, microbes that cannot spread to a new host learn to cooperate with the one they are stuck with.

But cooperation in society took a back seat with the rise of private property, the keystone of power. Historically speaking, the ability to control what's yours is a relatively new way of doing things. As farming-based societies grew up in place of hunter-gatherers, there arose the notion of "mine," rather than "ours" or even God's. In the Old Testament, humans were stewards of the earth, but because of the nature of ancient Hebrew we cannot tell whether it's talking about Adam's own progeny or the earth when God told him to "multiply and replenish." However, from what we have seen over the ensuing millennia, his progeny certainly have not replenished the earth!

All resources belong to God in that story. In most traditional societies they belong to Mother Earth, especially those that aid survival. But when men began to till the ground and domesticate animals, they learned how to gain power through accumulation. In what remains of the first written language, Babylonian cuneiform, most of the deciphered writings are about property lines. That was the birth of what we call Social Darwinism today, where the Babylonian god Baal, the archetype for the Voldemorts of modern day, was cut loose from the constraints of sharing resources for the benefit of all, making self-interest the norm and the quest for power the goal.

Was that a mistake? If it was, we are immersed in it and have no realistic way out. We do have many tactical measures to compensate for the erroneous hierarchy that naturally followed the rise of private property, but strategic measures elude us. Even autocratic attempts to eliminate private property in the Soviet Union and China ran up against the kulak's resistance (Russian peasants wealthy enough own farms and hire labor) and the failure of Mao's Great Leap Forward. Those attempts failed because collective interest must be balanced with self-interest. Both are valid pathways in evolution.

In the Mormon theology of my younger days, self-interest is even extended to the gods. In their explanation of the 'War in Heaven' mentioned in Revelations between Michael and the devil, the cause of the war was God's refusal to accept the devil's plan for us earthlings that would save everyone by eliminating free will. And, of course, the devil wanted the glory for saving everyone from the judgments of a jealous deity. While I am reasonably sure that the gods have found a solution to artificial hierarchies, likely centered in the combination of love with power that Reverend King describes, glory is a powerful meme, and self-interest is not far behind.

Self-interest is here to stay, so the best we can do is to follow Adam Smith and Alexis de Tocqueville, two great thinkers whose ideas influenced the development of American society, and add to self-interest the appendage they used *properly understood,* indicating the realization that well-being is a social issue—an individual's well-being is always contingent on that of their community. It brings us back to what both evolution and religion teach us about using power in combination with love, a natural and reasonable way of curbing the abuses that started plaguing humanity after the spread of the practice of accumulating wealth through private property. Much of what ails us stems from what's not properly understood, and next we'll look at a prime example.

IMPROPERLY UNDERSTOOD: IMMIGRATION

If properly understood means the recognition of our dependence on others in our community, *improperly understood* means putting yourself before the community. In the prequel to this book, we used the analogy of the warp and the woof, suggested by my granddaughter. It's something every good seamstress knows about, and using it to represent the fabric of society introduces the cosmic analogy of Indra's net as the foundation of the universe—it's the web of not just interdependence but also inter-existence, where everything exists in connection with and *because of* everything else. For our purpose, the warp and the woof is an analogy for the balance between self-interest and collective interest. Both are necessary for the strength of a fabric, and are meant to be in balance, but in our society self-interest is stronger than collective interest. It overwhelms cooperation and weakens the fabric. When the fabric comes under stress, it is more likely to rend and tear, and our society is under tremendous stress.

Evolutionary biologist David Sloan Wilson points out in his book on altruism that self-interest wins out *within* groups because we trust individuals in our group—even when their gain is our loss—but altruism wins out *among* groups because cooperation increases the group's fitness in the long-term. Cooperating with the group leads to more evolutionary success. The message about altruism is reinforced by psychologists looking at the results of their favorite game, The Prisoner's Dilemma, showing clearly that cooperation, not competition, wins in the long run. It's a lesson from evolution—not a belief, but a fact we should not turn away from—and the keystone of my cure for our present condition.

There are many examples of this imbalance between the warp

and the woof. Healthcare is one we touched on. Immigration is another example, and we can look at immigration policy to see self-interest driving the dysfunction. For one, stoking the immigration issue is directly profitable for the cartels behind the illegal transporting of immigrants; the immigrants don't have a better option in many cases, so it's in the interest of the cartels to prevent the implementation of fixes. But the real benefits flow to the politicians and media talking heads who build their careers around "the immigration problem." Historically, we could go back to biblical times to find examples of exploiting the issue, but in modern times we have political strategist Kevin Price Phillips and how his upbringing in ethnically mixed New York City during the 1950s gave him the idea to run political campaigns based on pitting ethnicities against each other. Richard Nixon took note and imported the idea as his "Southern Strategy" to win his 1968 presidential campaign by peeling away Democrat voters in the South who felt betrayed by the party's civil rights efforts, and the tactic continues to be used today despite the divisions it causes, the lies it spreads, the citizens and individuals it labels as *others*, and the many problems it spawns.

It's a variation of the divide-and-conquer strategy used in Machiavellian games of power, like in Nixon's War on Drugs. Which wasn't really about drugs at all, it was about attacking the groups seen as his enemies. Nixon's aid for domestic affairs, John Ehrlichman, revealed the truth to *Harper's* in 2016:

> We knew we couldn't make it illegal to be either against the [Vietnam] war or blacks, but by getting the public to associate the hippies with marijuana and blacks with heroin and then criminalizing them both heavily, we

> could disrupt those communities. We could arrest their leaders, raid their homes, break up their meetings, and vilify them night after night in the evening news. Did we know we were lying about the drugs? Of course we did.

But worse, perhaps, is that the tactics make such a mess of the political environment, and implementing fixes becomes impossible—not to mention the staggering number of people who went to jail for relatively minor crimes, tearing apart families and communities. Phillips built his political machinations around eugenics, considered to be a scientific reality only a few decades earlier. The mixing of the races was both criminal and believed to pollute the higher castes. Such memes, meaning cultural features or types of behavior that are passed from one generation to another, without the influence of genes, are not buried very deep—they keep popping up in one form or another, like in today's political campaigns that stoke the immigration issue.

Political gamesmanship gave us the toxic war on drugs and the toxic war on immigrants. Imagine if Donald Trump didn't have the immigration issue to harp on during the campaign in 2016. With no reason to "build the wall" on the southern border to keep out the "rapists and drug smugglers" he would have lost a big chunk of his appeal to people who thought of him as the strongman needed to protect them from threats that, truth be told, were largely nonexistent. One of his favorite stories during the campaign was about the caring woman who nourishes a sick snake back to health only to have it bite and kill her. It sums up his ruthless point of view that compassion only leads to abuse, an idea that cements into vulnerable minds the concept of *others* as threats rather than neighbors.

Remember when George W. Bush made immigration reform a major plank of his 2004 presidential campaign? Probably not. Fresh off his re-election victory, he tried to parlay his political power to push for reform in 2005, but the effort was dead on arrival in Congress. Fixing the problem would have been a 'shoot yourself in the foot' move for politicians who build power atop the divide-and-conquer strategy of stoking fear about immigrants. They gain power by pitting ethnic groups against each other, a lesson ingrained into our nation's history and resurrected by Kevin Phillips during the era of civil rights reforms.

On the other hand, people must eat, and who do you think picks the crops? The annual influx of immigrants is literally a lifesaver, and they do a job no one else wants to do. Many are from families who've been doing it for generations and asking for relatively little in return. When they stopped showing up to do that job, scared off by the threatening rhetoric and the congressional actions in reaction to their constituents' fears, millions of tons of crops rotted in the fields. Talk about shooting yourself in the foot!

While we must stop criminal elements from entering the country, we can't allow immigration decisions to be based on fear and influenced by people who stoke it to accumulate power. Like living organisms that rely on nourishment to live, living nations rely on immigration. Our job as individuals and as a nation is to know who to take in and share our bounty with—and how.

European nations are under strain from the many refugees they've taken in from Africa and the Middle East. Rapidly taking in refugees threatens the existing populations and opens the door to ethnic-based politics, reminiscent of Trump's story about the woman and the snake. We can't just open the doors wide to let in anyone, but they do need to be open. Otherwise, a nation becomes like a monoculture in farming. It suffers from lack of cross-pollination.

Forgive this comparison, but biological analogies are not inappropriate: Immigrants are like the excess food we store for future use. As they adjust and find their place in their new society, they become a resource that benefits everyone. But like eating strange food, the digestion process can be rough. It happened in Lowell, Massachusetts when Cambodian refugees flocked to the city after the Vietnam War. For two generations, they stayed in the proverbial pantry, apart from and unintegrated into the community. Then, trying to draw them into civic participation, the city decided to publish the minutes of official meetings in Khmer, the native language of its ethnically Cambodian citizens. The small gesture made a substantial impact. Immigrant participation in local elections rose, and the immigrant population felt increasingly part of the community. It's an example of the sort of back-door fix that pulls people—even seemingly strange people—together into a community. That action fits the strategy of a democracy far better than divide-and-conquer political tactics.

It is unfortunate that we don't find more places like Lowell, Massachusetts using innovative thinking to solve problems, rather than creating more of them like we've seen in Florida, Texas, and Arizona, where immigration policy is abused for political gain. Across the board, the dysfunction it causes grows worse. Pick an adjective like huge, immense, or enormous and pair it with "problem" and it falls short of capturing the truth of the situation created by political tactics. The crisis threatens our existence. The "American Experiment"—the creation of a free society governed by a unifying set of principles and ideas summed up best in the immortal words "life, liberty, and the pursuit of happiness"—may, when the final history is written, be deemed a failure if we don't do something to counter-balance America's self-interested individualism. That, and very possibly our future was seen by John Adams, who, in thinking largely about the French Revolution, wrote to John Taylor in 1814:

> Remember Democracy never lasts long. It soon wastes, exhausts and murders itself. There never was a Democracy Yet, that did not commit suicide. It is in vain to Say that Democracy is less vain, less proud, less selfish, less ambitious or less avaricious than Aristocracy or Monarchy.

The reasons behind Adams' sorry conclusions are many, but most of them have to do, as he implies, with the dominance of the warp's self-interest out of balance with the woof's collective interest. The unbridled quest for power is the umbrella for all self-destruction. To those on the left of the political spectrum, economic power is the most blatant threat, and for those on the right it's political power. And it's easy to see the threat of both. If the corporations win, we are led to a fascist world like that desired by leaders of the Wall Street putsch of 1933. If the left wins, the tendency is toward more socialism. But both lead to, and depend on, the power and the cancer of money in our system as they each paint the opposition as *others* and *dangerous*. That cancer is metastasizing throughout our society, sickening it top to bottom.

IMPROPERLY UNDERSTOOD: MONEY IN THE SYSTEM

In our comparison of nature with society, money is a conundrum since there is nothing in nature that functions as money does in society. In nature, cooperation ripples outward because it increases the niche of the actor and the system. Sometimes that causes a massive die-off, as happened when microbes learned how to make oxygen a few billion years ago; the oxygen killed off most of the anaerobic bacteria, but it opened the door for plant and animal life to emerge. The anaerobes moved underground where they continue to make the methane and oil we use for power and heat.

Money has a niche role in a marketplace. Just as expanding one's niche drives evolution as part of the fitness landscape, money acts similarly in a marketplace. It establishes a value on items and services, acting as part of the fitness criteria for failure or success. It also brings into the picture the possibility for self-interest to be *improperly understood.*

Which brings us now to how self-interest improperly understood combined with the corrupting influence of money in the political marketplace sent it into a death spiral. While money and politics have never been a good mix, the tipping point for our political system was reached when the Supreme Court's *Citizens United* decision supported the self-interest paradigm. The Court ruled that unlimited amounts of money could be spent to game the system. Many argue that our elections were always a part of the marketplace, but the decision destroyed any effectiveness of the market. The cost of elections prior to its enactment in 2010 was never more than $50 million. In the 2010 midterms, the cost quadrupled to $200 million, then mushroomed to over $1 billion in 2012, and in 2020 it topped $4 billion. If the marketplace is an accurate measure of value, our politicians are worth their weight in gold! And their corporate sponsors accept that, because their money buys influence, and influence buys greater ability to profit. Without that money, a political candidate has zero chance of getting elected, and when they do get elected, their primary job is not governing—they spend the majority of their time hitting up their corporate sponsors for "donations" to fund their next campaign. *Citizens United* created the ability for corporations to buy the country's political system, and it's a marketplace where only the richest can play.

Union wealth and power, which for decades flowed mostly to the Democrats who supported workers' rights, became the political target. In a move made to create the impression of fairness, *Citizens United* gave corporations the same rights as unions; they could use their corporate money and whatever their supporters would contribute, openly or as "dark money" (money from unknown sources—even foreign), to influence elections. But it's a disingenuous tactic because first of all, union money comes from its members—it's not "dark money." And secondly, it amounts to nothing compared to that wielded by corporations and industries. Unions have trouble coming up with a million dollars, while on the other hand there are a few corporate donors today coming up with a billion. In terms of time, a million seconds is about twelve and a half days; a billion seconds is 31 years.

The legal reasoning behind *Citizens United* is based on the conservative justices' concept of *originalism*—that we should try to think as our Founders did and apply it to the issues of the day. But that would mean we would have to dump a passel of amendments that made the Constitution a fairer and more just instrument for governing. Originally, only property owners could vote—and who controls more property than those owning and running large corporations? A good part of the added fairness and justice baked into the Constitution came about because of amendments added in response to slavery and the Civil War. The caste system is alive and well in originalist thinking, and it shows in the decisions made by the Court that support the elite classes at everyone else's expense, corrupting the marketplace that is our political system.

James Ho is an avid originalist federal judge on the Fifth Circuit covering much of the South. When some of their proposals were included on the ballot and rejected, he lamented:[8]

> Originalists are disparaged and destroyed. We're not merely wrong as an intellectual matter. We're not just disagreeing in good faith about the proper meaning of legal terms. We're fundamentally bad people who are just too extreme for polite society. We're mean spirited, racist, sexist, homophobic. We're just trolling or auditioning.

Those on the left see Ho's lament as an accurate description, and that corporate power is the primary nemesis, but the right sees it differently. From that point of view, corporate interests are trying to rescue our nation from abusive political power seen in all of the regulatory bodies present in the executive branch because the legislative, having been sold to the powerful interests earlier were not interested in limiting their funders. The problem, of course, is that they rely on an autocrat to get rid of the bureaucracy. The problem with power is that we need a different paradigm to manage it, something other than warfare thinking that fights power with more power in an arms race that ends up with nuclear options, and only increases the money flowing through the system. Our Founders did that by attempting to balance competing powers in government, and it lasted for two-and-a-half centuries, only to be overcome by the power of money.

We dealt with this problem in the Progressive Era when we got tired of robber barons and the wealthy controlling the strings of power. The government listened and began establishing agencies designed to control the abuses of the powerful. Much of that thinking is still alive today, but in 2010 the tide turned decisively toward financial power.

Taking a lesson from the originalists, one way of dealing with the corruption of financial power is to implement George Washington's suggestion to establish a citizen-to-representative ratio of 30,000 to 1. That would mean my county, population 32,000, would have its own legislative representative. Would he or she need a million-dollar campaign fund in a town that size? Is there anything in governing that an elected representative could not do online (where there is a record), with Zoom, or a telephone? With an office downtown, would he need to rely on a bunch of lobbyists to help him decide the issues, or would he listen to his neighbors? Better yet, since he is local, he could call on the community to form a task force to look at problematic issues and come to a consensus opinion. That's what Obama tried, also in 2010, in commissioning America Speaks, a Washington DC-based non-profit organization to gather groups to discuss issues that impact the lives of Americans. Despite the fear that the discussion groups were not representative—they actually were—and their conclusions about how to address many of the biggest issues faced by our nation were superior to what the partisan-locked Congress offered.[9] The aim of the community groups would be to find consensus. The aim of autocrats, here and abroad, working through our media, is to build and accentuate the cracks in our society. The focus of these local committees is to heal them.

With legislators doing that in their communities we could transfer the reins of government back to the people—and that is the point. The money-drunk marketplace of government would be relocated to our communities and sanitized, and the money deluging our political system can be made unnecessary by strategic actions that alter the fitness landscape. We'll have more to say about this later.

CHAPTER 3

Conscious Evolution

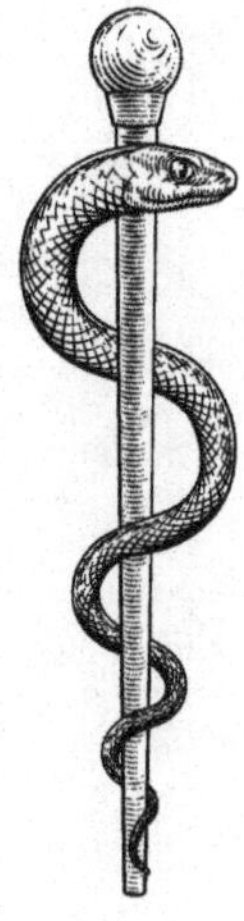

Paul Ewald is a revolutionary thinker about disease, as seen in his book *Evolution of Infectious Disease.* He opened the door to thinking of how to play with the microbial fitness landscape so that we can make microbes friendlier to us. The process he describes is essentially the same as Darwin's: mutation, selection, and reproduction. Mutations are random in nature, but today we have CRISPR—a technology that allows us to play with it. Selection is not random; it must fit into the environment—and Ewald shows us that it, too, can be played with, and done so in far safer ways than CRISPR. This is because we are familiar with the environment. The options for microbes are getting to another host, (virulence) or living with its current host in a friendlier way (commensalism). Ewald showed us that blocking transmission pushes the microbe to the commensal pathway. In other words, he showed us how by using window screens and bed nets to constrain the spread of malaria, and condoms to prevent HIV we can negotiate with microbes. We knew that doing so prevents illness, but we didn't know that it helps tame the microbes. And guess what? Our own physiological defenses do the same thing, and we can do it with glycans and their mimes. It's a new idea, a different way of seeing, one central to this book and its prequel, and one that needs reproducing, but with our defenses and glycans not being profitable the only ones doing the reproducing are those who understand the need for regular negotiation and see the benefits. If that is you, please share your experience with everyone you know.

Commensal mutations ultimately benefit us. The microbes become part of our biome, the three trillion microbes living with us that help us live better and longer. It's a revolutionary understanding of our relationship with microbes and the benefits of cooperating with them.

George Williams and Randolph Nesse, in their book *Why We Get Sick: The New Science of Darwinian Medicine* took a big step in the right direction by showing how the natural defenses of the body and mind, such as fever and depression, are normal and helpful ways of addressing underlying problems. In the first *Commonsense Medicine* book, we extended their idea to the defenses guarding the vulnerable openings to our body, the airway and GI tract. Now, we extend the idea of defenses further to our social and political worlds. Millions of years of evolution passed down their survival benefits to us through natural selection, and they can be seen in every aspect of complex living systems, from microbes to humans, and to the systems we design as humans. Traits selected in such a way are highly likely to be the best options available for fixing a problem and restoring equilibrium, our treasured homeostasis, in both our human and political bodies.[10]

Each of us can engage our microbial world to adapt in win-win ways just by keeping our airway defenses optimal. And we should be able to do similarly with our hostile political foes; we just need to better understand what to take in and what to leave out.

This is the premise of my prescription to make America healthy again: use our understanding of evolution to build a fitness landscape that guides superior and friendlier adaptations. But the walls built around beliefs and centuries-old memes—especially the beliefs that self-interest *improperly understood* is more important than community interest, and that evolution is somehow contrary to religion—are making the body politic vulnerable in much the same way that the human body is made vulnerable to infectious disease. These beliefs are easily transmissible since they satisfy the egos of many, but they do contribute in big ways to our illness, both individual and collective. An ancient illustration hints at how.

Glaucon was Plato's brother, and he posed a thought question to Socrates. He asked if there was ever a man with the moral strength to deny the advantage of Gyges ring, which made the wearer invisible, of using it to satisfy all his animalistic appetites. It was a good question, and we are told that Socrates delayed in answering. And when he did answer, he did not really answer the question. He pointed out that the self-interested and indulgent person became a slave to those appetites, and he pointed to a well-functioning community and advised following what makes them work. And what makes them work is the application of natural selection in a community where both self-interest, in smaller groups, and altruism, in larger, more diverse groups, play their parts. People would rather be cooperative and make all boats rise together, rather than be mired in a winner-takes-all competition.

Seeing how xylitol optimized our airway defenses reinforced my understanding of defense medicine and opened the door to a wider use of defenses. I had used oral rehydration (ORT) for my patients with GI problems since I first began practicing fifty years ago, and the medical literature is now full of information about its use with cholera as an alternative in poor countries that lack IV therapy. I saw it as a way to keep our back-up GI washing defenses from killing us with dehydration, like cholera does, and to save a ton of money—estimated at a billion dollars annually—if used in place of much more costly IV therapy.[11]

Defense medicine recognizes the critical role played by our physiological defenses—both primary defenses, with no symptoms, and secondary ones, with symptoms that tell us the body needs extra help. Symptoms such as fever, runny nose, and diarrhea are the body's way of helping itself, but antipyretic drugs for reducing fevers, and antihistamines for reducing runny noses, suppress the symptoms at the expense of crippling those defenses. Anti-diarrheal drugs interfere with the body's natural defense of washing the GI tract, consequently enabling pathogens to gain a foothold. These actions are taken in the name of balancing symptoms, a central tenet of humoral medicine, where the practice of bloodletting to balance symptoms of inflammation comes from, and while bloodletting has perished, the thinking behind it is alive and well—but dead wrong, pun intended.

Inflammation is the body's defense for both injury and infection. Its primary symptoms—redness, swelling, pain, fever—prompted doctors who practiced humoral medicine to respond by bloodletting, just as today we use drugs to combat them. While bleeding people with injuries did little harm, especially when the injury was splinted or treated, they were more likely to die if they had an infection. That's what Pierre-Charles-Alexandre Louis, a founding father of epidemiology, found when he looked at hospital records of those with pneumonia in the 1820s. The defense response of inflammation brings all of the blood-borne defenses to fight the infection, and bloodletting, and the shock it induces, cripples that defense. But the practice was so ingrained that some doctors were still bleeding patients a century later during the 1919 flu pandemic—a reason why so many died. The reason it was so ingrained was due to their focus on symptoms. All of the symptoms of inflammation listed above are eliminated by the redistribution of blood seen with the state of shock that follows the loss of blood. You could literally watch your patient's symptoms resolve as the bloodletting continued. Today, if your focus is balancing symptoms, we can do that easily with drugs, but make sure the symptoms are not defenses.

The understanding I gained about our natural defenses allowed me to see over the walls of the medical paradigm and foresee the end of humoral medicine's hold on the minds of physicians who believe that relieving suffering by using drugs to balance symptoms—symptoms caused by our defenses telling us they need help—is the best approach. And it gave me crucial insights about how to practice a type of medicine that works with nature instead of against it.

Since the time of Francis Bacon (1561-1626), doctors have thought it their highest duty to relieve suffering.[12] Today, we have an arsenal of medical weapons to accomplish that, but much of it comes at the cost of short-circuiting the body's natural defenses, and I believe it does much more harm than good.

At the heart of humoral medicine is a philosophy based on correcting the imbalances seen in the symptoms, but microbes offer a different approach. When they sense a threat such as a decrease in population density—like after being hit with devastating antibiotics that carpet-bomb the biome—they basically take a vote (known as quorum sensing) to decide whether to act or not. Action is ramping up their mutation rate to counter the threat—leading to our problem of antimicrobial resistant organisms. Another option, also following quorum sensing, is for some of the microbes to self-sacrifice to build a protective biofilm matrix around the colony. In both cases they are wiser than us; it's the threat that is addressed, not the symptoms.

The same thing happens in the immune system when exposed to infecting organisms. It responds by repeatedly mutating until finding the best antibodies against the invader. That's why our lymph nodes swell up in response to an infection—it's where all the mutation happens.[13] Problem is, mutation is random, not planned out, and most of these mutations end up in the garbage pile of uselessness, which is why our lymph nodes swell up when we have an infection. Successful mutations in the immune system become memory cells with specific antibodies against specific types of infection. Those mutations are remembered by the body and ready for use in case of future exposure, but for the most part they are not inherited. Instead, each person has to go through the process of building their own immunity. But recently researchers have shown that snippets of DNA left over from ancient viral infections help build protection against modern ones.[14]

A bit more specificity is needed here because the molecules needed in this identification are the glycans[15] on our cell surface, specifically those on our immune globulins. So, the mutations are all about which glycans go where, and there are billions of possibilities with the twelve glycans. If the ancient DNA codes are for the immune globulins and their glycans, then some of our adaptive immune system is indeed inherited.

We need to be more thoughtful about how we apply what we learn from microbes about fighting infection. Paul Ewald showed us how to constrain microbial mutations by altering the fitness landscape. The virulence pathway is where the microbes solve the problem by finding a way to increase their spread—virulence is all about transmission. Once established, the third part of evolution (reproduction) becomes important, and microbes are much better at it than we are. They can double their population every four to twenty minutes, and when it occurs after a beneficial mutation, microbes put it in a plasmid and share it with any other organism needing help. The commensal path, on the other hand, is taken when the path to transmission is blocked; successful microbial mutations then become less deadly to the host. It's the cooperative path. The microbial organism adapts to be less virulent. Cholera and HIV are two examples Ewald cites where blocking transmission with clean water and condoms triggers commensalism.

A better example is found in a dental study done on young school children in Belize showing that chewing gum sweetened with xylitol prevents tooth decay, but the researchers were not sure how it did that. They knew that microbes eat the sugar in our foods and subsequently produce acids that cause tooth decay; tooth decay is a type of infection, but how did xylitol prevent the production of acids? For a long time they thought it was because xylitol is a five-carbon sugar that many microbes cannot digest; microbial indigestion can cause them to concentrate on other things, but the study in Belize found that assumption to be wrong.

The first study lasted two years, and compared xylitol gum with sorbitol, which xylitol won. Five years later, a second study, with no xylitol administered in the interim, gave everyone a big surprise: The permanent teeth that grew in while the children were chewing the xylitol gum had 95% fewer cavities than their neighbors in the same mouth that erupted after the initial study ended. If microbial indigestion was the reason for the benefit, tooth decay should have returned to its normal rate when they were not exposed to xylitol. As one of the authors of this study explained to me, "the only explanation for this result is that either the bacteria are not there any longer, or they have changed to not make the acid."[16] Subsequent research found evidence for both, but the bacteria that remain are clearly adapting to circumstances by taking the commensal path. *The point here is that this change was an evolutionary one that was stable and had dramatic benefits to the person—it's something we need to learn from and use.* And the most likely reason for this beneficial result is that the microbe behind the decay's preferred glycan docking site on our teeth can be blocked when xylitol is regularly in the environment. As with Ewald, the message from xylitol is either shape up (be commensal) or ship out (virulence not practice here). Either way it's a win-win.

Sometimes, microbes co-exist with humans in a parasitic relationship, but over time they adapt to not just live and let live but to aid us like little elves working behind the scenes. Our body's surfaces, both our skin and the tracts within us needed to eat, breathe, and reproduce, are covered inside and out with microbes adapted to live cooperatively with us. Most of them are greatly beneficial and live, technically at least, outside our bodies. That's because the lining of our inner tracts are made up of the same family of epithelial cells that our skin is covered with. It's an "inner skin." The epithelial cells that are inside us are interspersed with cells that make mucus, and the mucus is filled with the glycans, the same ones that also cover our cells and that are the preferred docking sites for microbial invaders. It's the mucus with all its glycans that provides most of our defenses in the places where we are open to invasion from viruses and other microbes. But an equally important part of these inner defenses is comprised of our commensal microbes, what we know as the human biome—and our health and development is very much tied to its health and development.

It's almost too simple. We've discovered what makes microbes tick and how to make them friendlier to our health, and with some serious work and research we are likely to make many more discoveries. But since xylitol is a food, not a drug, don't hold your breath. No pharmaceutical research money is going to flow that direction. There's a bigger picture, too, that includes lessons we can learn from microbes that apply to our health and the health of communities and societies and nations, and we turn our attention there next.

EVOLUTION, COMPLEXITY, AND THINKING

Microbes have been evolving for at least four billion years. In that time they learned how to cooperate. They learned that sometimes cooperation is even better than survival.

From our human perspective, evolution is seen simplistically as what helps us to survive better by not marrying a relative, or racehorses faster by wise breeding, but it's not a matter of winners and losers in competition. It's a matter of evolutionary fitness with the environment and the ability to reproduce more. It can also be viewed as a drive to increased complexity, where the women have a distinct role seen in the increased genetic diversity of primitive matriarchal societies. Cross-pollination leads to both healthier seeds and healthier and more complex societies.

It's like integration in math—every time we integrate, we add a new constant and variable, and boost the power of every other variable in the equation. After two or three of these integrations you end up with a very complex equation—just like life. That's what happens with a successful mutation, and it's been going on for a long, long time. In the human world of ideas, the same thing happens but over a much shorter time span.

Evolution of the nervous system is part of that process of increasing complexity. Current microscopic studies have found evidence of embryonic brains in fish dating to more than 400 million years ago, before land animals even began. And fish developed the schooling response to avoid predators beginning around 250 million years ago, enabling them to instantly cope with a predator targeting them for its dinner. Then, around 50 million years ago, reptiles, the first animals to develop an organized, rudimentary brain, inherited this response to threat and modified it, adapting it to the reptile's more solitary lifestyle and adding a new level of complexity. The response originates in their eyes, ears, or noses and is sent to their rudimentary brain where it triggers a rapid response—fighting, fleeing, or freezing—that saves their lives. Paul MacLean, one of the leaders in looking at our neurological evolution, described the triune brain. The primitive midbrain—what he called the reptilian brain—came first. It controls our breathing and is where the startle reflex comes from. On top of the midbrain is the limbic brain, which evolved in combination with extended relationships needed with dependent offspring. And the cortical brain, with its two hemispheres, was fully developed in mammals and primates, but the midbrain, what he calls the reptilian brain, persisted.

Humans inherit both the rudimentary "lizard brain," and its limited options for response, as well as the higher structures that evolution added to it, structures that allowed us to give it a scientific name—the *acute stress* response. But despite the added complexity it has not added any other options, we are still stuck with fight, flight, freeze, or flock. The reaction of my fellow traveler to my mention of evolution is illustrative. He *fought* against accepting my idea, took *flight* from further conversation, *froze* his thought processes, and flocked with the many sharing his views. They are instinctive, protective responses against the danger of an idea seen as challenging his beliefs.

Humans added another layer of complexity and another "f" to the list of possible responses to threat or danger: "fawn," as in fawning over someone, seen in particular among domestically abused women when told to *just treat him nicer and things will get better*. I don't believe this to be a true alert response handed down to us by nature because it is not instinctive. I know of no examples of fawning in nature—submission? Yes, but being nice to your oppressor? No! It's more of a response to abusive power than to the existential threats that trigger the acute stress response. However, fawning is a protective response to threatening situations, and it's important to our discussion for the reasons we're about to discuss.

A major problem with the stress response is it bypasses the rest of the brain, particularly the higher functioning parts, leading to inferior tactical choices that may not be in our strategic interests. The midbrain controls fundamental processes like breathing and escaping from existential threats, driving tactical rather than strategic decisions, and it becomes a problem when, for example, it makes us think that arming everyone in response to violence in society is a good idea, thus creating more violence. Solving the problem is the role of the higher brain, the human cortex, but the stress response bypasses it. We react instead of thinking, and that's a big problem.

Reducing existential threats is one huge benefit of civilization, but civilization produces new threats, like the threat my friend felt about evolution because of his religious beliefs. The alternative strategy of cortical thinking is not an option when the primitive brain is in control, and anything that does manage to seep through to your head when feeling threatened is likely to be a justification for actions taken in response to acute stress. You hear about a mass shooting, for example, and feeling threatened, you buy a high-powered weapon, justifying the danger you've added to your home because of the presence of that weapon by saying that you're better off being armed. But by a wide margin, the statistics clearly show that having that gun in your home is a much greater threat. The lizard brain strikes again.

With existential threats where life hangs in the balance, the acute stress response works well. The ability to instantly fight or flee or flock or freeze could make the difference between survival or death. But when the threat is to our ego or world view, we need to take a breath, or several—deep ones—and let them out slowly. That's a simple way to say "hi!" to your cognitive brain, where wiser decisions are born. Indeed, lizard-brain thinking not only alters our relationship to the outside world where the threat originates, but also the development of the brain and body; the hormonal messengers of the stress response cause our muscles to get bigger and our brains smaller.

Another element added to evolution by our brain development is that our relationships have become deeper and more widespread. We can thank the limbic system for that. It sits atop the primitive brain and governs our emotions and behaviors in relationships. It adds sympathy and other complex emotions to the repertoire of higher animals, and for humans it makes us value our important relationships and abhor the thought of someone close to us dying. Relationships soften us in a way, perhaps due to the influence of religions that teach us to help the poor and the handicapped, in support of the commensal path.

Of course, in retrospect the complexity of the development of the nervous system and brain can be seen in simple evolutionary terms of variety, fitness consequences, and heritability, but since complexity comes with self-destructive potential, evolution should not be credited yet. Microbes don't have the benefit of higher thinking, yet they can and do make decisions to move toward commensalism, and when they increase their mutation rate they avoid the potential for self-destruction by making only part of the colony participate, a fail-safe maneuver. Paul Ewald notes that the inability to get to another host prompts them to move in this direction. It's not like they carefully think things through, it's just that the cooperative pathway opens when the virulent one is closed, making the virulent pathway a dead end. This is a crucial insight we can learn from evolution to apply to us as a civilization. We need to block the virulent elements from infecting the rest, and we'll get into specifics later.

Ease of transmission is a critical part of virulence, and it can be blocked. Paul lists all the methods we have for doing this and promoting commensalism—like isolation, bed nets, and condoms—and he shows that when put to use, diseases like cholera and HIV become less virulent. But he ignores the physiological defenses we all have that evolved with us to cope with our infections. They apply the same pressure, and unfortunately that tendency in thinking leads to ignoring the other side of health care—the side of defense, which has been getting the short end of the stick dating back to Louis Pasteur's time. Defense medicine offers key insights and practices in our search for answers to make America healthy again. That's our next subject.

EVOLUTION AND CIVILIZATION: DARWIN'S INFLUENCE

As explained earlier, the fundamental parts of evolution are change (mutation or idea), fitness characteristics (how it fits into the environment, what I call the fitness landscape), and reproduction. And these principles really apply everywhere there is change.

Interfering with transmission (virulence) and thus promoting commensalism are examples of how the fitness landscape shapes success. The success of the virulence pathway requires an open host whose defenses are less than the microbes' adherence ability. This allows the microbe to spread to others, but it is specific in who benefits—and it's not the host.

We need a better way to think about this problem. While we are the dominant species on this earth we are beginning to understand that the microbes are perfectly capable of killing us off. They need a lot more respect than what we have given them since Pasteur put us on the war path.

The international service group Rotary uses their Four-Way Test to define what good service to our fellow humans is, but it is just as applicable to microbes, as well as every other creature we share this earth with:

1. Is it the truth?
2. Is it fair to all concerned?
3. Will it build goodwill and better friendships?
4. Will it be beneficial to all concerned?

While this test was designed for humans, with our current understanding of our co-existence with microbes it is just as applicable there. One can easily see how it constrains our choices in defining what fitness is. It can no longer be what most helps the individual, instead it must help all involved. It's how to steer evolution in a win-win direction. It also illustrates how fitness landscapes can change. The truth today is not what it was yesterday or a millennia ago. Biologically, there are no differences between people to justify hierarchy or caste. As our indigenous people tell us, we are partners on this earth with many other species: we need to be fair and just delegates for *homo sapiens* to the congress of the species. Adam was not given ownership; he was given stewardship.

Mutations and ideas happen, and they are mostly random. Whether they are helpful or not depends on time in the genetic realm and how it fits into the physiological landscape. In the memetic realm it depends on seeing an advantage and building the fitness landscape to help it succeed. Xlear provides an example here of what happens when the landscape is adverse. Our current landscape for drugs is constrained by the FDA and *de facto* excludes safe foods with drug effects. *De facto* because that manufactured landscape was justifiably built to protect the public from snake oil salesmen; efficacy was added in the 1960s, requiring far more expensive testing on people. But as the cost of drug approval rose, foods were caught in that net with no way to recoup the cost of FDA 'drughood'. Their grocery store prices can't raise the same as approved drugs can to repay expenses. But Xlear certainly satisfies the Rotary test: it works; it helps the user; and it's inexpensive. When I first heard about xylitol, it was used to prevent tooth decay. Then I read that its use there also prevented many ear infections. But many of my patients with ear infections were too young to chew gum. The study said it worked on the microbes; they live in the nose; I put it there. When I found out how much better it worked when spayed in the nose I knew I was onto something, and despite being unable to tell people what it does, annual sales have grown 10% since it came on the market. That reproduction rate comes mostly from people sharing what it does with their friends and family. It's up to all of us to find out what works, lest we ignore the powers of evolution.

Darwin recognized change in all the many specimens that he had, and he saw the beauty of natural selection. It fit nicely into his analytical framework. But once you add the fitness landscape as a constraint for success, and our ability to manipulate it, the analytical framework is no longer sufficient. Natural selection is a simple process, but inserting a fitness landscape that can be defined by self-interest removes the simplicity. We are left with solutions that emerge, then we must find out why, and where the benefit is. *Qui bono*, who benefits, leads us to those self-interested, and is often the most fruitful tool in parsing, but skilled manipulators can often use decoys that alter the public's focus away from the real intent.

Parsing was the problem Darwin had in trying to understand the evolution of civilization; he got stuck at the level of human relationships and sympathy, the human versions of commensalism. There were just too many elements in the equation, and the tools for understanding those elements were not at hand. He could not see, for example, the cooperative communication that drove the evolution of early communities, nor, as their complexity grew, how a division of labor was needed.

We have better tools today. The analytical tools helpful in the physical sciences are being replaced by those looking at what works in the far more complex social sciences, and while they are certainly not perfect, they are helpful. A humorous example of it not working is from Bill Easterly's summation of the attempt by the Commission on Growth and Development to determine the reasons for economic success:

> "After two years of work by the commission of 21 world leaders and experts, an 11 member working group, 300 academic experts, 12 workshops, 13 consultations, and a budget of $4m, the experts' answer to the question of how to attain high growth was roughly: we do not know, but trust experts to figure it out."[17]

The problem with economics is that it is still embedded in the hopeful predictability of the physical sciences with all of its mathematical precision. They have not yet opened to the realization that economics is more a part of the life sciences where its complexity defies analysis.

Understanding Life and Social Sciences is what we are getting at here. They are about *us*, and just as humans cannot be analyzed—despite Freud's attempts—neither can the 'sciences' that look at other complex systems. One has to see what solutions emerge and try to figure out why. And the best way to gain this understanding is to learn the fundamentals of evolution and use them to help us learn what and why something works. The secret behind economic progress may be simpler than the experts would have us believe, like making beer from three ingredients: barley, hops, and yeast. Thousands of varieties of beer can be made from them. *Three* is the border of complexity. The interactions of the sun, earth, and moon is another three-body problem. So is the female cycle of estrogen, progesterone, and testosterone. Modeling these on a computer gives answers, but it's nigh impossible with a pencil and paper. Shifting the fitness landscape is how one plays with the elements. More specifically, it involves making the fitness landscapes favorable to growth, which can be done in a variety of ways. Learning to see what works and who benefits is key.

Ultimately, the answer to what works is altruism: consideration of others. In the self-centered game of survival of the fittest, you can gain an advantage through selfishness at the expense of the individuals you operate with, but that approach actually lowers the fitness of the group when compared against groups that are altruistic. Or, thought of another way, the selfishness epitomized by Social Darwinism produces short-term gains at the expense of a civilization's long-term health. *Time* magazine has estimated that our neoliberal top-down support for the self-interested has transferred fifty trillion dollars from the bottom 90% to the top 1% over the last twenty years.

A better goal is to maximize the evolutionary fitness of the society, not just the 1% at the top, and that means we should focus on building altruistic societies. It's a dawning realization in the wake of a period where the self-centeredness of neoliberalism has dominated our thinking and understanding. Altruism is the better evolutionary pathway than the one we've taken, the one based on the ingrained belief that "survival of the fittest" justifies cutthroat competition as the basis for building a society. Darwin actually made the opposite argument.

In his writings about evolution, Darwin used the term sympathy because empathy as a term did not come into existence until 1908. If it had been in use during Darwin's time, he most certainly would have found in it a better way of describing his thinking on the subject of the evolution of civilization. The same goes for economist Adam Smith, whose book *Wealth of Nations,* was based on his earlier book, *A Theory on Moral Sentiments,* which argues that human sympathy is the keystone for a healthy society. Sympathy is a feeling for others, like when you sympathize with someone's plight. Empathy describes one's feelings, not just *for* the other, but *as* the other. Empathy is what one person uses to understand the position of another, to walk a mile in their shoes, and like altruism it is more of an emergent process. Altruism spurs us to consider the welfare of others equally with our own—as in the Rotary test. It's reasonable to assume that Smith, like Darwin, would have found empathy to be a better term for describing his thinking and argued in favor of altruism as the moral guiding force of decision-making in a market economy—it's the basis of Smith's *invisible hand* that guides the moral marketplace to an ever better future.

The science of Darwin's time also did not have access to study in detail the microbial world where cooperation is the norm, but he saw hints of it in the natural world and tried to communicate that evolution is much more than a simple mechanical process like natural selection. The environmental constraints seen in the *fitness consequences* that frame this second step of evolution open the door to seeing all organisms able to determine what to take in and what to leave out. It's a complex world of living organisms that is driven by some measure of consciousness that, instead of being localized in the brain, is universal. Life is consciousness, and consciousness is life.

Humans take pride in their thinking abilities, which supposedly set us apart from all other living things, but that idea is being destroyed by researchers finding memory building and conscious behavior in animals with no brains. Cells stuck together in a laboratory work together to accomplish a task, and plants do the same:

> Indeed, the very act of living is by default a cognitive state.... Every cell needs to be constantly evaluating its surroundings, making decisions about what to let in and what to keep out and planning its next steps. Cognition didn't arrive later in evolution. It's what made life possible."[18]

This concept will open a new paradigm for those studying the life sciences. For one, mutations may be purposive and not random. Mutations in the centers of our lymph nodes are specific in searching for just the right enzyme, to add just the right glycan, in just the right place, to build just the right antibody to combat an infection. And for two, Heisenberg's *uncertainty principle* tells us we cannot know both the position and the momentum of a fundamental particle, and that particle can choose to be either a wave or a particle depending on how we ask our questions. Those behind the cellular studies have no problem extending consciousness to answer these conundrums. It not only made life possible, but it's also what brings the physical world into being. The nature of our questions will shift in very interesting ways.

Our purpose in this book is to see how we can make ourselves and America healthy again. America is seen here as a large organism made up of individuals just like our bodies are made up of all our individual cells—and we too need to do better at what to let in and what to keep out, but in this case it's the ideas that we let in, not the immigrants. The whole cannot be healthy without the parts, and many of the parts in American society see themselves as insider-groups where selfishness beats altruism and ruthless competition affords them greater fitness within their group. Evolution wired our brains to follow primitive survival influences, but as we got rid of existential threats our lizard brains were too powerful to get left out, so we transferred ego threats to the existential realm. That keeps many of us in the threatened mode of thinking, in fight-or-flight mode, but when we take the time to think about it, we can choose a different path that leads to the altruism of making everyone healthier—that's the difference between the warp and the woof.

Later, we will propose specific ways of accomplishing that objective. First, we need to figure out where and why we went wrong, then we'll see how defense medicine corrects a major mistake of our preceding scientific thinking.

A WRONG EVOLUTIONARY TURN

Anthrax is largely a disease of herd animals, and it was a big problem in the 19th century. We thought we had it licked until global warming thawed out some infected reindeer in Siberia, sparking a local epidemic, proving that it is still a problem. It was the focus of Louis Pasteur's experiments with sheep, goats and cattle, and his findings are the reason why we have germ theory and our war on microbes today. In 1881, he developed a vaccine for anthrax using a method that made the bacteria weaker and unable to cause disease. A simple way to do that is to grow them in the lab. When we do this, they rapidly lose their glycan coating, which is what enables them to hold on to us. But they can also get it back with a taste of nature.

Pasteur had no idea of how our three trillion resident microbes help us, but we know a lot more now. When he showed the world that invisible organisms (germs) are behind our infections, he lit a fire in our lizard brains. The existential threat made us think that our only rational option was to fight. While we knew there were lots of microbes in our mouths and feces, the understanding we have today about the role(s) of the human biome had to wait until the early part of this century. Microbes are the titans of life on this planet, the original and only inhabitants to have lived here for two billion years as they both adapted to and changed the earth's environment to make it more complex. Our war with them is a cosmic one that, if Reza Aslan is correct in *How to Win a Cosmic War,* we should never have started in the first place.

And despite what we believed to be true, we really did have another option, but it was a fringe one. Claude Bernard argued with Pasteur that the soil where the microbe is planted—our bodies—is just as important in determining who gets sick as the microbe. Bernard is honored today as the father of modern physiology; he understood the working of the body, and some about the defenses we have gained by natural selection that put a lid on our infections. Bernard and Pasteur were both right, but without a clear definition of our defenses Bernard lost out, both then and now.

The fitness landscape of medical progress has been framed in Pasteur's warfare mode, and it has not changed yet. But we are trying. Previous books have explained how xylitol works, and the prequel to this book is a clear challenge to the prevailing paradigm. It explains our airway defenses all the way down to our mucin glycans that act—like xylitol—as decoys for microbial binding.

Whether we like it or not, our healthcare system took a wrong turn, and it could be about to get a lot worse for all of us. The World Health Organization (WHO) predicted that antimicrobial resistant organisms will kill *ten million people annually* by 2050. Five million this year, ten million by 2050, and at that rate of doubling it won't be long until the threat engulfs us. This is an existential crisis that competes with global warming, and it's all due to a wrong-headed tactical decision to fight microbes instead of learning how they tick and encouraging them to live cooperatively with humans.

The warfare mentality isn't solving the problem, not in medicine nor in world affairs. Moshe Yaalon, Israel's former Minister of Defense, summed up the problem with warfare—including Israel's own Palestinian problem—with his statement: "In our tactical decisions we are operating contrary to our strategic interests."[19] The lizard brain strikes again. We feel threatened and in response we go to war. But as we are learning from the rise of antimicrobial resistant organisms, recurring epidemics and unwinnable wars, that mentality only makes things worse, in part because its only options are tactical, they are made in the midbrain, not the strategic cortex. Think strategically and the better choices become obvious, but they aren't as popular nor as profitable and therefore aren't given due consideration.

For well over a century, our healthcare system has focused on fighting microbes and blamed bad personal behavior for illness. Surprise! Things got worse. Neither has it helped the research community to focus on using advancements in technology to parse out the minutiae of the body's genes and proteins rather than focusing on helping people. Relying on analysis to understand complex systems is also a wrong turn, and that misunderstanding affects the fitness landscape.

The moment of realization for former head of mental health at the National Institutes of Health, Dr. Tom Insel, came with the help of an audience member during a question-and-answer session at a presentation he was giving. "You don't get it," said the person in the audience, to which Tom asked, "get what?" Expressing a common point of view among people who work within the system only to see it fail the people it's supposed to serve, the audience member clarified his statement: 'you're telling us about the molecules in the paint as the building is burning down.' Insel saw the truth, quit the NIH and began focusing on the *people's side* of the equation. That's where he could do the most good. NIH and other big institutions focus on analysis down to the minutiae of the chemicals in the paint, burning away countless amounts of money and energy. It's the analytical approach we learned from Newton, but it doesn't work for truly understanding complex living systems because they are networked—eliminating analysis as a tool. That requires a big-picture perspective that includes the people affected.

That kind of change in thinking is needed if we are to have any hope of keeping the WHO's prediction from coming true. Microbes evolved to cope with most any type of threat, including whatever new antimicrobial tactic we can come up with. We are not able to analyze ourselves out of our war with them. That war was the wrong turn, but it has taken us nearly two centuries to realize it.

Claude Bernard countered with a commensal approach of bolstering physiological defenses. Paul Ewald added insights on how to get microbes to behave, and now it's clear that the fitness landscape determines success or failure. Aid the immune system, bolster defenses against infection, give people a healthy environment to live in, and most health problems take care of themselves. That's basically what Bernard meant when he told Pasteur that the soil also plays a large role in who gets sick and who doesn't, and it's the essence of my brand of defense medicine. When working optimally, our defenses exert commensal pressure by blocking the transmission of microbes, and it benefits us and the microbes. This understanding corrects the wrong turn.

Taken further, commensalism could be the new "*ism*" to govern our world by showing us how to live together. Adjusting the fitness landscapes in our societies to promote commensal adaptations could lead us all to a friendlier world where we survive as our *homo sapiens* ancestors did—by cooperative communication.

Learning to live cooperatively with microbes helps us survive and develop better, live longer, and share the benefits through natural selection. Same goes for learning to live cooperatively with each other. If you think about it—and please do—you will see that humans can and do sometimes follow the commensal path in evolving our cultures. The creation of the European Union exemplifies this thinking. While digging out of the aftermath of the Second World War, European leaders devised a way of trying to stop such destruction from ever happening again by banding together to live cooperatively. When Ireland's "troubles" led to nothing but violence, the Good Friday Agreement offered a commensal resolution. And both worked very well.

On the other hand, wherever the warfare mentality wins out, the problems only get worse. Israel took that approach with the Palestinians and now finds itself with no choice but to continue escalating the violence to the point of committing genocide. Kalev Sepp, a history teacher at the Naval Postgraduate College in Monterrey, California, examined more than one hundred examples of insurgencies around the world and authored the monograph, "*Best Practices in Counterinsurgency*." His key insight shows us that using only military force against an insurgency usually results in failure (as we are seeing with Israel) but address the underlying reasons driving it and there's a good chance of winning.

Kalev was impressed when we shared with him the parallels between his insurgencies and infectious disease. The lesson is universal. There is a better way. For example, the various opposition elements to India Prime Minister Modi's Hindu-centered government took a step in this direction recently when they pooled their resources to win enough seats in their parliament to spoil Modi's majority. The leadership in Israel needs to hear that message. It's the same lesson we need to learn from our war with microbes. There is a better way.

Commensal resolution versus more virulent hostility—which is proven to work? That's easy: Sepp's findings are clear.

Mutations happen in bacterial cultures in response to changes in their environment. In human cultures, ideas are the agents of change, but change is tough, and tougher still when the best way to profit is through the old ways of doing things. Entrenched interests epitomize the old ways. They are the profiteers from outrage, conflict, and warfare at all levels, and their self-interest takes highest priority. My experience with asthma is a good example.

After finding that our xylitol nasal spray stopped asthma, I began a study to prove it, but then the hospital and clinic where I worked closed, and I returned to working at local emergency departments where such research is not an option. But I also began trying to find someone to continue the research. Researchers I approached expressed interest and support, but no action. Local societies were no help, either, but the wives talked, and my wife, Jerry, heard that the reason for the lack of action was the fear among doctors that a simple and inexpensive fix for asthma would be bad for their business. It became clear that an asthma researcher who actually cured the condition would be out of a job.

Things have not changed much from a century ago when a group of New York pediatricians petitioned the mayor to stop a school centered hand-washing program initiated by Dr. Sara "Jo" Baker to cope with epidemics of typhoid and cholera. Their reason was the lack of sick children was hurting their practices! She wrote in her biography that it was the best affirmation she could have received.[20]

Self-interested, *improperly understood* thinking dominates our culture, making the commensal brand of thinking a tough sell, but it's a crucial one because otherwise as a society we will keep making the same wrong moves. The tug of war between virulence and commensalism is the same as that of self-interest, where fitness is measured by power and profits, versus cooperation, where it's measured by personal and collective health. Cooperation is how we live together in increasingly larger communities with their social and economic pressures, but truth be told, it's always been the better way. We don't choose it because as a society we got sold on a big lie known as Social Darwinism.

SOCIAL DARWINISM AND EVOLUTION

Both pathways, the commensal and the virulent, are included in the rubric of evolution. The change occurs in the power structure of the environment. The fitness characteristics are defined by competition, and reproduction is conferred by power, so the criteria of evolution are satisfied. The problem is, in nature there is no power structure. Dominance, sure, but power over another is slavery, and the one example found in nature of ant species enslaving other ant species reeks of anthropomorphizing. It's like saying that homo sapiens enslaved the neandertals.

But Social Darwinism is all about power, and that type of thinking is based on a terrible misunderstanding of Darwin's natural selection. Social Darwinism thinks of natural selection as competition, summed up in the 'survival of the fittest' mantra, but natural selection is based on beneficial mutations gradually spreading throughout a population through reproduction. Social Darwinism was *not at all* what Charles had in mind. Nowhere does he justify the survival of the fittest mentality and the rule of society by the most powerful individuals and institutions. They argue that their high status grants them the right to the lion's share of resources, but that's chutzpah. Making the argument takes *gall.* Plus, it's just wrong.

Soon after Darwin published *On the Origin of the Species,* Herbert Spencer, who coined the term survival of the fittest to describe Darwin's ideas about nature, expanded the idea of fitness to include the survival of the elite in our societies, a social spin on Darwin's theories. Spencer ignored the evolution of human caring as the basis for the advancement of civilization and replaced it with the competitive mantra of *winners and losers.* Of course, Spencer's idea appealed to the elite as a justification of their position in society, and it continues today, but it has nothing to do with Darwin's evolution. If our focus is on evolutionary health for our community, we need to focus more on Darwin's view of natural selection, and while virulence is a part of that picture because it benefits the individual (microbe or person) we need strategies that follow the commensal pathway of win-win, rather than Spencer's competitive focus on win-lose.

To see where the Social Darwinist view leads in society, consider Newt Gingrich. He grew up wanting to be a zookeeper, enchanted by what he thought of as the savagery of nature, and in politics he brought with him that same winner-takes-all mentality. His brand of politics spawned the nastiness and dysfunction in politics today, according to Thomas Mann of the liberal Brookings Institute and Norman Ornstein of the conservative American Enterprise Institute in their book, *It's Even Worse Than It Looks: How the American Constitutional System Collided with the New Politics of Extremism*. It tells you something when two big names from opposite ends of the political spectrum agree like that. Rational debate has ended, the extremes own Congress, and governing is impossible, and it's mostly to blame on Gingrich's brand of no-holds-barred politics and the Republicans who bought into it.

Maybe it would have been different if Gingrich had a better biology teacher in school to teach him that nature doesn't work that way. Things are shared in nature, especially in the microbial world. But in the human system, the drive for profit makes sharing at best a quaint notion from Social Darwinism's point of view. In my world, this fact of life pushed me to patent my nasal spray. That way I could profit from it, but the real profit is found in what it did for the health of the millions of people who use the spray. My main reason for patenting it was my fear that the pharmaceutical industry would beat me to the punch. It's in their interest to bury innovations like Xlear that aid natural defenses and prevent health problems, and indeed they are trying.

It was in my interest to make my innovation as widely available as possible, and to that end I freely share the formula: put about a teaspoon (5 grams) of xylitol in a 45 ml bottle of saline nasal spray. Allow about an hour for it to dissolve completely. When you spray it in your nose, look at your toes. The reason is because our nasal passages do not go upward, they go backward, so bending the head forward allows the bottle to be upright, where it makes a spray rather than a stream. Inhale briskly so that the spray is distributed more to the back of those passages, which is where most of the problems originate. By the way, recent studies have shown that erythritol, another sugar alcohol, is better than xylitol at blocking the adherence of the H1N1 influenza virus, so if you want to cover that base as well use a half teaspoon of each.

Pecuniary interest is nothing new, but the commodification of healthcare made it much worse. The argument in America has always been that health care should be in the marketplace, and commodification was seen as a step in that direction. But in doing so, the consumers in the market—us, the patients—were replaced by other players that have no interest in cost efficiency, or even our health, despite what they claim. Insurance companies being the primary payers in the healthcare market obscures just how much out-of-pocket costs are rising along with the big profits for healthcare companies and all the middlemen who've got their fingers in the pie. The medical model is based on illness and disease, and has been for more than a century. The sicker and more diseased a population is, the more opportunities there are for profit. Gerald Posner's book, *Pharma: Greed, Lies, and the Poisoning of America,* is an eye-opener that traces the greed, lies, and poisoning of America back to that industry. But the commodification of healthcare is more than 'pharma'. The profit incentives of commodification are institutionalized throughout the system, driven by giant companies that call the shots and collect the profits. The inevitable conclusion is that we are sick by design, and if not by design then at least by a wrong turn.

Our acceptance of Social Darwinism's paradigm exerts a great deal of pressure on how we see and perceive. Dr. Todd Rose, co-founder of Populace, a think tank committed to ensuring "that all people have the opportunity to pursue fulfilling lives in a thriving society," thinks the Social Darwinist view of the world is a *collective illusion.*[21] In his book by that name he offers the results of a survey asking people about their view of success, giving them two choices:

A. A person is successful if they have followed their own interests and talents to become the best they can be at what they care about the most.

B. A person is successful if they are rich, have a high profile career, or are well known.

Ninety-seven percent of the 5,200 respondents chose A, but ninety-two percent thought that their neighbors would choose B. 'B' is therefore a collective illusion, but it's just as congruent with Social Darwinism, competition and the virulence pathway as 'A' is in following one's bliss and finding their niche in the world. But I would wager that there are many who choose A because it is congruent with their vision of B.

Michelle Dresbold is a psychologist and expert at handwriting analysis, and is known for her analysis of presidential signatures and what they indicate about their style of leadership.[22] Donald Trump's signature, she says, describes what we see as the warp: "workaholics who are sharp-minded, competitive, angry, hostile, aggressive, determined, driven, fearful, rigid and uptight"—and who know (or think they know) all the answers. They are competitive men, businessmen, and the wealthy and powerful of both genders; they tend to view those characteristics as desirable. It's no surprise then that Dresbold's audiences, made up of those types of people, tended to see them as being positive and share them in common. But others—women, teachers and university professors, certain politicians, and everyone who values empathy and the woof of cooperation—see them as negative.

The people in Trump's camp share the characteristics Dresbold described, but they take it to the next level. Trump is seen by most, and accurately in my point of view, as a narcissist. His community is one of tribal narcissism, the tribe of white Anglo-Saxons who feel threatened by everyone who isn't like them. They are more interested in their own survival than the health of their community or the welfare of those they do business with. The resulting polarization threatens our democracy, and in the long run it threatens the survival of society itself.

In evolution, as in the weaving together of the fabric of society, equal strength is necessary, but Social Darwinism promotes the strength of the warp at the expense of the woof. The balance is found in altruism and community. Self-interested Social Darwinism is the warp fringe in our social fabric, the negative aspects of virulence and the infection of our minds and hearts. It's suicidal for a society when the health and welfare of one's community is essential for a good life, or even for survival. And the thing is, very rarely is it better to put self-interest over community interest, even for the people who benefit in a society like ours where Social Darwinism has taken hold, because we are all passengers on the same sinking ship. We could say that Social Darwinism is a collective illusion, but the powerful financial interests holding that view have made it real—in accordance with the Thomas rule—and it is real in its consequences. The fact that we put choice B off on our neighbors may give us some hope to correct the problem.

Collective illusions have power because they are simple to understand; they are not complex. We have discussed complexity a bit earlier and will do more so later, but understanding that we are complex, and that our societies are as well, is a key part of their management. In mathematics complex equations do not have simple answers; their answers are in the form of attractors or basins of interest—and these have real counterparts in human society. Basins of interest are like paradigms, mental constructs we build and live in; and they are like foxholes that keep us safe from outside dangers. They create the proverbial bunker mentality. The entrenched interests, like those that own and control our healthcare system, use their enormous wealth to build high walls to protect their interests, and deep foxholes to avoid thinking about the consequences. And they drag the government into their bunkers, to the point of passing off liability to the government for problems stemming from insufficiently tested vaccines; it creates an impenetrable barrier to change no matter how dire the situation. The only way to rescue them is for those outside the foxhole, i.e. the public, to drag them out.

We do that by showing them there is a better way, for them and for all.

OFFENSE AND DEFENSE IN MEDICINE AND SOCIETY

Offense medicine is our current paradigm. It's the foxhole for the entrenched interests in healthcare, for the standard ways of thinking, and it not only focuses on attacking microbes, it attacks aberrant symptoms and lab tests as well. Rather than looking to see if the bothersome symptoms are the body's immune system doing its work, doctors view symptoms as aberrations to be suppressed, mostly with drugs. Lab tests showing deviations from the norm are used to justify unnecessary treatments and over-prescription of drugs. The mentality behind offense medicine blames health issues on microbes and personal behaviors. While there are many unhealthy behaviors that need attention—smoking, alcohol abuse, poor diet, etc.—the focus on them ignores the social matrix of health.

For instance, Surgeon General Murtha reported that loneliness has the same-sized impact on health as smoking. But there's no drug to fix loneliness or any other social issue, so there's little interest from the medical-industrial complex in doing so.[23] Blaming the patient helps no one, but it does give excuses to ignore the complex social and behavioral factors in personal health.

Attack, attack, attack—it's how the big profits are made. It dominates our thinking not only in medicine but in government and society. We have a problem—attack it! So, we declare war—on microbes, on cancer, on drugs, on terrorists. But talk about limiting your options. They say that when you only have a hammer, everything looks like a nail. We hammer away at our problems and end up creating more of them. That's our reptilian brain in action.

And what does it accomplish? In metaphorical terms, we become the nail. We get hammered, making us sicker, an argument made by Williams and Nesse in *Why We get Sick.* Hammering the body with unnecessary drugs and treatments to suppress evolutionary defenses of fever and depression cripples those defenses, and it's a likely reason behind our decreasing longevity. With life expectancy actually decreasing despite the increasing sophistication of our medical treatments, the disparity is a bright, flashing red sign that something is badly amiss.

Defense medicine is a new paradigm giving us a new way of thinking. It looks at balance and equilibrium in new ways that include helping our defenses so they can be more effective at preventing microbial infection. It expands on Paul Ewald's idea of blocking transmission externally to include blocking it internally by optimizing our defenses. It expands and extends the hygienic practices that began during the 19th and early 20th centuries that were responsible for the dramatic increases in life expectancy we experienced.

Life expectancy has been worsening in America ever since the medical-industrial-complex took root during the 1950s. During the previous century, life expectancy rose at a rate of three years per decade. After 1950, around the time cold pills came out and commodification began with the use of health insurance, it dropped to two years per decade. Around 2010, when the Affordable Care Act (Obamacare) empowered the health insurance sector at the expense of physicians and decisively changed the balance of power, the rate of increase halted. After ten years of zero increase, COVID and pain killers were blamed for our recent decline in longevity, but that's the opinion of people stuck in a basin of interest. To acknowledge the real reasons would require prying open the eyes within our healthcare system to the fact that it's a big part of the problem.

Take the Institute of Medicine, for example. Founded in 1970 as part of the National Academy of Sciences, it aims to improve healthcare, but its recommendations come from people within the basin of interest of people—mostly highly successful doctors whose interests are first and foremost in improving their business models. So they make recommendations such as Surgi-centers to cut the cost of surgeries, and for HMOs to refocus on prevention, that nibble at the edges rather than take a real bite. Their 2001 book, *Crossing the Quality Chasm*, acknowledges the chasm between what we pay for and what we get. Twenty years later the chasm has become a canyon, and the Institute of Medicine has become the National Academy of Medicine, but its vision remains parochial. Adding a few biologists could perhaps help them focus on the wider issues of health care, and while they're at it they should listen to Linda Gorman from the Wisconsin Policy Research Center, who wrote about the problems caused by third-party-payment.

By changing the medical paradigm from offense to defense, we can make a huge leap not only in life expectancy but in overall well-being, and it couldn't be simpler. Defend instead of attack. When the body is out of balance, support its natural defenses. ORT supports the cleansing of the GI tract by keeping the body's fluid tank full, so when you have diarrhea, reach for a tall glass of ORT (a mixture of sugar and salt in water) rather than an antidiarrheal pill. The pill may help you to feel better, but the associated risk is that the cause of the problem may be microbial and the more time it spends in your body the more opportunity it has to make itself at home. Xylitol is another support for the body's defenses. It optimizes the cleansing of the respiratory tract by keeping it wet and functioning optimally. And equally important, by interfering with microbial adherence. ORT and xylitol aid the body's defenses instead of suppressing them, and they work where the body is most vulnerable to microbial invasion that leads to infection.

The blocking of microbes is a revolutionary way of understanding balance. It is a new paradigm. And it's no longer just about the individual person and their microbes; it's about balance among both people and microbes. It's not win-lose; it's win-win.

Microbiologist Bill Costerton taught us about biofilms, the safe houses microbes build to protect themselves from antibiotics and other threats, and gave us the insight that the glycans on our mutual cell surfaces mediate the contact and docking of microbes to their target cells in us. He proposed creating drugs to interfere with this process, not realizing that sugar alcohols are structured to do this. Sugar alcohols are often based on the sugars that are in the twelve member family of glycans: xylose is a five-carbon glycan; N-acetyl glucosamine and mannose are six-carbon gylcans; and their sugar alcohols are xylitol, sorbitol, and mannitol. The alcohols have one more hydrogen atom, which breaks a bond in the molecule making them flexible and even better able to fit into the complementary glycans on the microbe to prevent docking. They thus carry the invading microbe to our immune system where the process of building immunity is begun.[24] Costerton also points out that this does not threaten the well-being of the microbe and therefore does not trigger resistance. Instead, a microbe docks with the sugar alcohol and is eventually washed out of the body. Sugar alcohols are like decoys—talk about a great defense!

Bill wrote his article in 1978 and it's been cited more than 2,000 times in the scientific literature, which is really almost negligible for the information it contains, so it's not surprising that nothing has been done about looking for agents that interfere with microbes like sugar alcohols do. Research sponsored by Xlear Inc. at the Antiviral Research Center at Utah State University shows that sugar alcohols can block adherence in the manner suggested by Costerton nearly fifty years ago. But when the Xlear company told the country about it in a press release, they were sued by the Federal Trade Commission for false advertising. Stopping the war on microbes and the pandemic and preventing millions of deaths with a simple-but-revolutionary food blocking mechanism is not on their radar.

It couldn't be clearer that change is needed. Competition has won over cooperation. Our ecosystems need changing. *We* need changing. Answers are staring us in the face and have been for decades, but they are ignored.

The first thing you'll hear from the people in their bunkers is discouragement about how much the changes will cost, but it's a red herring because they easily pay for themselves. Implementing ORT over the common practice of using an IV, for example, is estimated to save *one billion dollars* in the US annually. Optimizing our airway defenses would virtually eliminate respiratory infections and the pandemics that spread via our airways, saving trillions of dollars by avoiding a pandemic on the scale of COVID, while virtually eliminating allergies and asthma. But look at the downstream effects as well, such as the special education needed to help kids with language and learning problems stemming from not being able to hear. Their chronic ear infections early in life, when the brain is optimally fit for learning the sounds that make up our languages, are the major reason for their learning disabilities. The infection actually begins in the airway, where xylitol works its magic. Remove that problem along with the others through the simple-but-effective defensive strategies proposed in our prequel and our healthcare costs would likely return to something we could afford.

Cooperation—it's the key strategy behind defense medicine. Cooperation sidesteps resistance. Just as Kalev Sepp showed us that the key to countering an insurgency is through addressing underlying problems, defense medicine teaches us how to stop insurgencies in the body from microbes that turn virulent. Both medicine and society can be revolutionized by simply respecting the opposition and looking deeper than the surface for answers, by negotiating and cooperating rather than acting like might makes right. It's not how nature works, despite what Social Darwinism would have us believe.

WHERE'S THE BALANCE?

Nature works by balancing competing interests, and examples of it are everywhere. Take giraffes and acacia trees. Giraffes must eat, and acacia trees, like everything in nature, want to survive and thrive, but eating too many leaves from one tree can threaten its survival. So nature gave acacia trees a defense, a bitter alkaloid the tree elaborates when too many of its leaves are eaten. The giraffe gets the message and moves on to another tree. Many varieties of plants make alkaloids to persuade pests to go elsewhere, and many alkaloids are toxic in high doses. Like antibiotics, too much can be deadly.

Similarly, as every farmer knows, obliterating the pest population now creates an imbalance that leads to more resistant infestations in the future. Industrial farming uses monoculture in the name of efficiency, but it breeds virulence. Pests can take hold and wipe out entire harvests. Whether you want to call it spreading or transmission (the medical term for the same process) it's another reason why balance is needed.

Bacterial resistance is triggered by quorum sensing. Bacteria in a colony release a messenger molecule when they sense their numbers decreasing. A tipping point is reached and the colony's defenses spring into action by forming a biofilm, a protective 'skin' around the colony. With that defensive matrix protecting the colony it takes 50 to 100 times more antibiotic to get inside, which is enough to kill the patient.

Whether through overuse of antibiotics or monoculture, the result is imbalance. Nature then restores balance in ways that cause big problems for people.

Collective defensive action is the woof aspect of bacterial life. When an antibiotic tears through a bacterial colony, quorum sensing triggers the formation of biofilm and ramps up the mutation rate to collectively defend itself.[25] Bacteria in biofilm can cause infections, and the infections may be chronic and recurring. Many ear infections are due to biofilms. They recur because the bacteria stay inside their safe house while an antibiotic is present, then exit once the coast is clear. The infection returns, the person goes back to their doctor and is prescribed more antibiotics, and the process starts over. It's nature's defense mechanism, and it works very effectively.

Biofilm came into play in the case of my wife Jerry's dry eyes. Her eye doctor inserted plastic blocks in her tear ducts to increase available tears, but one of them got infected and it recurred after treatment with antibiotics. I informed her (uninformed) doctor about biofilms, and he removed hers. Problem solved. Another friend was not so fortunate. His biofilm was likely on a dialysis tube which no one thought to change. He died due to antibiotic-resistant microbes. Many older doctors are not familiar with the problem and need to be encouraged to read up on it instead of just prescribing routine antibiotics.

As I made these discoveries, I used our xylitol nasal spray on a niece with asthma, who likely suffered from a biofilm in her sinuses. Her healing episode came after two weeks of regular nasal spraying. As her mother was washing her hair, something broke loose in her head and she gagged and vomited and finally got rid of it. Her mom said it looked like tissue, and wondered if her daughter blew out a chunk of her brain! Six months later, my niece was playing basketball and doing gymnastics with no asthma. Turns out, in addition to washing microbes out of the airway, xylitol has an unhooking effect on biofilm as well. It's been confirmed *in vitro* (in the lab) by the Center for Biofilm

Engineering at Montana State University.[26] I believe my niece confirmed it *in vivo* (in a live person).

Quorum sensing in bacteria is a collective action process, and if you look hard enough you can find similar processes in human physiology. The rampant increase in antibody production in the germinal centers of our lymph nodes during the early stages of infection is likely triggered by a quorum sensing mechanism. And the cytokine storm that follows the destruction of lung tissue by SARS-CoV-2, which is almost invariably fatal, may also be triggered that way.[27] Steroids given to seriously ill COVID patients may prevent it by turning off the immune system, but administering them early is a mistake because the immune system is still trying to cope with the virus. A similar trigger is suspected to be behind the uncontrolled growth of cancer cells.

The immune system also works through collective action by recognizing the difference between what is native to the organism and what is foreign. Called the *sense of self,* it is the key action of immune system function. The glycans covering our cells—the same ones that form the bonds between our cells, and that microbes hijack to begin an infection—are the key components. Blood type, for example, is determined by the glycans on the ends of the chains extending from our red blood cells: fucose is type O, N-acetylgalactosamine is type A, galactose is type B, and acetylgalactosamine and galactose together make type AB. These glycans play a central role in our immune system and how the *sense of self* functions. The immune system senses and decides how to respond, and it will attack with antibodies if it senses a blood type that's different from the body's—a good reason to make sure you get the right type of blood during a transfusion.

Glycans are on the front lines of the immune system, and we

must be very careful about tinkering with them. They are much smaller than the proteins we target for research and manipulation. They are highly specific, working behind the scenes and undetected by our sophisticated tests, and just because they can be tinkered with doesn't mean we should. Through their variety, glycans tell our cells where to go and what to do. It's akin to a language for cells, but we are only in the earliest stages of learning it, and we need better understanding. Which is why these mimetic molecules should only be used externally. Most are not readily absorbed, and we need to keep it that way, but, as explained earlier, both the airway and the GI tract are lined with epithelial cells like those making up our skin. Using sugar alcohols in this way is what negotiates the win-win. Nature's balance is too easily disrupted by our tinkering—we need to keep it outside the body.

MICROBES AND GOVERNANCE

It's fascinating to think how our bodily systems and governmental systems mirror each other, and how language expresses this relationship, like when we say that a nation's collective group of citizens is its *body* politic. Take voting—could quorum sensing teach us something about holding better elections? Microbial communities use a quorum sensing to determine when to respond to threat, and a quorum in governance is the minimum number of members of an assembly or society that must be present at any of its meetings to make the proceedings valid. We could apply that lesson to elections by making the results valid only when a high enough percentage of voters participate, or a law is valid only when enough of us agree. People and governments are complex systems where evolutionary principles apply.

One of the things Bill Costerton noted in his article discussed earlier was that the microbes that were regularly studied in our many laboratories did not have a glycocalyx. They were not complex, they were homogenous, there were no strangers to mix with. All microorganisms found in nature have a glycan coating. Diversity requires a way to recognize and communicate with the other, which is what the glycans provide. What we have in society that is comparable is the cooperative communication that made our species successful.

In Catholic Ireland, many of its diverse citizens had a problem with their Constitution proscribing abortion, so they formed a citizens' committee to study the issue. The committee could not reach a consensual decision, but agreed in principle, and proposed a ban after 12 weeks and gave it to the public. The public agreed. But try that in the US and see what happens—in our partisan atmosphere, a compromise agreement is caving to the enemy. The media are divided, the think-tanks are divided, the people are divided. But in states where the citizens can initiate legislation the voters have agreed with Ireland. In practice, it worked with Barack Obama's America Speaks program of citizen discussion, which left a better track record for reaching consensus than Congress's.

The microbial world teaches us that collective action is never partisan. Take biofilms, for instance—they are composed of many different species of bacteria, and even include viruses. Quorum sensing represents them all. Beneficial mutations are shared across the board. We could apply that sort of nonpartisan action, too, but it seems to only happen when we are under a common threat, like after Pearl Harbor and September 11, 2001. We all pitched in to help. But it's back to business as usual after a threat recedes.

The problem with only coming together when under duress

is it drives acute stress responses, such as fighting and flocking, and overreactions like the military response after September 11 driven by tactical decisions that are not in our strategic interests. If the individual or the state takes a deep breath prior to deciding, a strategic solution is more likely to emerge, one where consent and consensus are essentials for decisions that affect everyone.

Consensual decisions demand that everyone is heard. Different points of view are understood and honored, and a consensual path found for moving forward. So how do we model the microbial world when making decisions? We argue to learn. Movements such as Occupy Wall Street used this approach, instead of arguing to win, the consensus-killing, dominant method in polarized societies. The signers of our Constitution acted consensually. They didn't agree on everything but were satisfied with its compromises, realizing that it was better than the status quo, and that ratification by the states stood little chance unless they acted as a unified body.

A unified *body*. It's no coincidence that so many terms used in governance are also used in physiology. In a representative *body* of government, we do best when we make decisions in the name of the whole, same as in medicine, but these days the whole is mostly ignored. Instead, the loudest, most partisan voices win, the needs of the whole are ignored, and money provides the megaphone for pushing priorities to the front of the line. It's like in medicine when we pay attention to symptoms and lab tests but ignore well-being. Under the current paradigm, we don't listen to the body. Instead, we force it to comply due to the louder voice of money. It's like arguing to win, forcing compliance instead of listening and addressing the needs of the whole.

Symptoms are akin to complaints and voices of dissent from some members of the body, and it is detrimental to override them.

Take the case of a woman whose gallbladder acted up. It voiced its unhappiness through pain. She sought medical help from three different doctors, and they all said to remove it surgically. Her test results, though, did not show her to be in imminent danger. The ducts were not blocked, and the organ wasn't infected. She decided instead to listen to what it was saying to her, finding a correlation between the pain it expressed physically and the pain she was feeling emotionally. She found personal meaning in the word *gall* and the function of that bladder to secrete bile. Bile also means bitterness; an emotion one can have difficulty "digesting." She found an alternative, diet-based course of treatment, and soon her gallbladder was happier.

Its complaints could have been 100% due to diet and not emotions, but the point is she saved the organ by listening to it. Surgical removal is the offensive approach, the more convenient and profitable approach than the alternative of patiently listening and carefully working through a patient's history and current circumstances to find the source of their trouble. Instead, we pretend that body and mind are totally separate, which we can blame on the philosophy of dualism. Making decisions in a vacuum doesn't work in medicine, and neither does it work in governance.

Listening to the body's point of view is a much better approach than forcing it to comply, yet our paradigm in medicine *and* in governance is to force compliance. Ignore dissenting voices and complexities. Might makes right is easier to implement than the subtleties of working with our problems creatively to solve them, yet we repeat the same mistakes by imposing our might and breeding resistance, costing us more in the long run. Then, we say, *gee, maybe that wasn't such a good idea*, but before long we repeat the mistake because we have not changed the paradigm. We need only look at the US invasions of Vietnam and Afghanistan for examples of how the Goliath US military suffered death by a thousand cuts from seemingly insignificant and weak resistance forces. You'd think that we would know better based on our experience in Vietnam, but no, we rushed into Afghanistan and made the same mistake. Again. Are we making that mistake in our approach to microbes, presuming them to be weak and defenseless, and not realizing that organisms that can survive for *billions* of years can outlast us? Despite how obvious the answer is, we're getting no closer to ending our warfare with them. Instead, we double-down on the same costly mistakes.

Negotiating an end to this war may mean the difference between *our* life and death, but it won't change until we make warfare unprofitable—both the medical kind and the military kind. Arms races benefit only the chosen few leading them, but they are costly for the whole. It's another reason why our medical paradigm is killing us and must change, and soon. The chances of recovery may vanish.

The message is loud and clear: It's time to follow the example of microbes for how to respond as a whole. With quorum sensing, a small-scale shift triggers a big one in the organism. In economics, Malcolm Gladwell calls it "the tipping point," and the same basic idea applies to cancer. After the tipping point, things spiral out of control. That's where we are today. The final direction of the shift is still to be determined, though. We can tip it in a favorable direction.

In healthcare, it's easy to see when the tipping point led to decline. Healthcare spending accounted for 5% of GDP in the US in 1960. Today, it is approaching 20%, a 400% increase. The chart below shows the US increases in comparison with other countries.

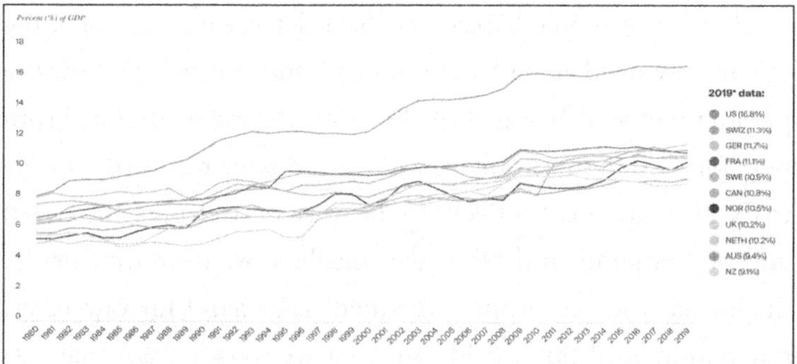

Notes: Current expenditures on health. Based on System of Health Accounts methodology, with some differences between country methodologies. GDP refers to gross domestic product.
* 2019 data are provisional or estimated for Australia, Canada, and New Zealand.

Data: OECD Health Data, July 2021.

Source: Eric C. Schneider et al., *Mirror, Mirror 2021 — Reflecting Poorly: Health Care in the U.S. Compared to Other High-Income Countries* (Commonwealth Fund, Aug. 2021).

What are we getting in return for so much spending? Singapore spends 5% of their GDP today on healthcare, the same as the US in 1960, and their system is one of the best in the world, according to the Bloomberg Report. For quadruple that price the US system delivers less, ranking far lower than Singapore. Copying their efficiency could save us $3 trillion annually.

To make America healthy again, we must begin there. The numbers tell the story of a healthcare system that exists first and foremost to generate obscene profits. Obscene self-interest like that does not belong in medicine. It does not belong in society. And it is making us sick.

The inefficiency of the US system is a problem, but profiteering is *the* problem. It puts 'we the people' on the table as the patient on life support, at the mercy of a system with deep pockets where $3 trillion disappears annually. The profiteers are not going to do anything about it, so it's up to us, the people, to act strategically by addressing the problem so clearly before us. The time is now in our nation, and now is exactly when we need to learn how to use defense medicine as an innovative disruption, as well as the tools of complex systems, to fix ourselves inside and out.

For fixing us on the inside, we have defense medicine. For the outside, we need government, society, and culture to follow the paradigm of well-being at the heart of defense medicine. From here forward in this book we will start looking outward for how to fix what ails us collectively. In the spirit of Asclepius, the Greek god of medicine, and other wise healers, we have the correct diagnosis, and the proper treatment is at hand for ourselves, our nation, and our world. But first we must accept that our system is broken. Look no further than our medical-industrial complex. Look no further than the self-interest thinking behind the belief that a person can do whatever they want to with the profits they earn, especially when it means that one person's gain is a big loss for another. Look no further than the thinking that makes it okay to hold self-interest above community and society, supposedly Darwin's idea, but no, it's just an excuse for selfishness. Look no further than the imbalance between the warp and the woof.

The warp path of evolution is valid when it follows a mutation or an idea that provides benefits as it spreads by natural selection. The benefits stay with the individual and all of us on the receiving end, a truly "trickle down" effect. Natural selection is a long road to travel for benefits to spread throughout a population, but the alternative is what, an autocratic decree? The problem with a decree, a forced change, is it bypasses the vetting process offered by natural selection. It looks beneficial at first because it offers quick fixes, but too often it doesn't hold up to testing. Testing takes time. It takes input from all voices that have a stake. Bacterial colonies learned its value long ago, a big reason for their survival. The picture of a healthy America, both individually and collectively, is one of mutation (change) percolating up though the society's natural selection process of recognizing and embracing solutions that restore balance.

Unfortunately, there's no interest in correcting the imbalances created by allowing the autocrats of the business world to dominate the system. That leaves us with the only other option of hoping for an "innovative disruption" or "creative destruction" that Clayton Christensen and Joseph Schumpeter see as the beneficial change, added to the system, that moves the paradigm to a new strange attractor. It's what we hope this book does. That disruption must come from outside the system, from innovative ideas that benefit the community, but the real force of change comes from the people. Their acceptance of an innovation drives the disruption—it's how the marketplace is supposed to work. And the people must have an understanding of the problem, a sense of meaning that comes from working together, and the control needed to resist the temptation of tactical, short-term responses over long-term strategy. These markers follow Aaron Antonovsky's ideas for how to measure health, and we will explore them in more depth in the next chapter.

Nature showed us how to make America healthy again and gave us microbial communities as an example to follow. The seeds are planted for innovative disruptions, found in the ideas of scientific thinkers who see the same problems in medicine and society that I do and want to do something about them. We now turn to them for answers.

CHAPTER 4

Looking for Answers

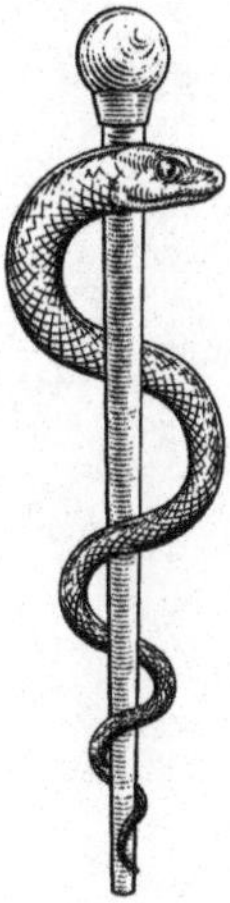

Our political structure is unraveling, and even though I am not a psychiatrist, unraveled patients get my attention as well. The problem for both is often a confusion of values, and that is also the diagnosis for both healthcare and the nation. We have chosen the wrong fitness landscape—that of profits rather than health or evolutionary fitness—to measure the success of our ideas and actions. The treatment is to replace the elements of that landscape with the healthier criteria that Socrates encouraged Glaucon and his followers to search for in healthier communities.

We determine the criteria through emergence in society, not through analysis or think tanks or committees of experts. Criteria emerge because they are shown to work through the consensual decision-making in a transparent marketplace environment, and through that process we found the following eight criteria:

1. The need to balance power.
2. The Wilderness Rules.
3. Analysis vs. emergence.
4. Counterwill—commonly called blowback, the instinct in all living systems to resist outside control—and the other side of the coin, cooperation.
5. The Prisoner's Dilemma game, used in psychological experiments exploring selfish vs. cooperative behaviors and the resulting fitness of each group.
6. The findings of both Daniel Kahneman and Jonathan Haidt on how our thinking is divided into reflexive and cognitive systems in the brain.
7. The discovery of the elements of resilience in family therapy and health.
8. Elinor Ostrom's ideas on how to rescue our social commons, the community pool of resources.

These ideas follow the wisdom of the microbial world and apply it to the political world. We will now plumb each one for what it can add to our understanding. Then, we will incorporate these ideas into our thinking and return to the subject of making America healthy again.

BALANCING POWER

Balancing power is an ancient concept, and the rules for achieving it originate across both time and space. Today, and for the past two-and-a-half centuries, we have had the Constitution and its rules for balancing power, most of which came from the European enlightenment figures of John Locke and Jean-Jacques Rousseau. But unknown to our Founders, their ideas likely originated in the conversations of the Baron de Lahontan with a Wendat chief Kondiaronk, which were published in 1703 and made their way to Rousseau.[28]

The Baron brought those ideas to Europe, from the minds of 17th century Native Americans to 18th century European intellectuals, and they made their way back across the Atlantic to the people forming the new American government. Would our Founders have better appreciated the natives if they had read Lahontan as well as Rousseau? If so, perhaps they would have done more to ensure that governmental power remained localized, where individual integrity is easier to ensure, and counterwill is minimized by giving people real ability to control their lives. The Hurons were not part of the Haudenosaunee Confederacy (also known as the Iroquois League), a group of Indian nations that formed a confederation for common defense as early as the 14th century. In fact, they were enemies, and even went to war. Local freedom is not necessarily shared with other tribes. That's the value of a League where tribal barriers are reduced by allegiance to a larger body.

The 14th century is also when Ibn Khaldun wrote the *Muqaddimah* (an early account of Islamic history), about balancing power and what makes a working government, and about the need for "asabiyya," translated as meaning social solidarity, group cohesion, and social contract. He describes a system where rulers recognize that their power comes from their people, and act accordingly. Khaldun saw the principle of asabiyya emerge as he looked at the rise and fall of several Arab states and noted that group cohesion is not only strongest in small groups, it decreases as societies increase in complexity.[29]

Nearly two thousand years before Ibn Khaldun, Confucius saw the differences in power and taught that maintaining order meant properly following rules about relationships, especially between the powerful and the weak, with preference always given to the weak. It's the relationship between a father and his children, and between a ruler and the people. The Mandate of Heaven, a Confucian doctrine that justifies power given to just rulers, granted the weaker people the right to overthrow those in power who failed to adhere to the expected benign and helpful behavior. It's fair to say that many of today's leaders fail that test.

There is another tool for balancing power that has escaped nearly everyone, and it is both simple and powerful. The Haudenosaunee Confederacy has an unwritten constitution that's been in place for more than seven centuries, and it has worked exceptionally well for fostering peace and cooperation. At the time of America's founding, it was the only known example of such a union in the world, and much was borrowed from its unwritten constitution in creating ours and finding ways to combine disparate interests. No one knew anything then of the tripartite government in what is now Moldavia, and with powerful neighbors and no protective oceans it didn't last long enough to be an example.

Another problem with our founders was their view of women. Despite Abigail Adams' plea to John to not forget the ladies, the Founders did exactly that. Even women of New Jersey, who had the right to vote in 1776, lost it after ratification of the Constitution.

And by ignoring the women, they lost a choice bit of balance seen in the Iroquois League: the clan mothers could impeach the chief. They called it dehorning, since wearing a horn was a symbol of being a chief. That lends to a good analogy because our abusive leaders would be hog tied if they did not have access to the horns of media to use in their service. Professor Bruce Johansen shared a 1989 letter from John Kahionhes Fadden, a Mohawk artist, describing a longhouse meeting where a dehorned chief who had been a charismatic leader and eloquent speaker could not resist the temptation to address the group:

> Anyway, at one point when all of these people were gathered, ...many benches deep with a lot of people standing in the doorways, and some outside craning their necks and cocking their ears to listen to what was going on, the "de-horned" former chief couldn't resist the temptation of that audience. He stood to talk to the gathered people, and, as you know, a "de-horned" chief isn't supposed to talk, and for sure no one is supposed to hear his words. He was able to get out about two or three brief sentences before he was abruptly interrupted by a slicing voice from

> the women's end of the Longhouse. She was a clan mother, and standing less than five feet tall, she made it quickly and abundantly clear that this man could not speak anymore. He had lost that right by abusing his former position. The six-foot, two-hundred-plus pound "chief" snapped his mouth shut, sat down, waited about a minute or so, then quietly, with his head kind of low, left the Longhouse. Now, as I see it, that's feminism.

And from a rational point of view there are few, as a class, who have a better understanding of when a man is bordering on abusing his power than a grandmother. This group of elderly women needs more empowerment instead of just 'a place for mom.'

Our cherished national governmental structures are time-honored and designed to balance power, but the powers have outflanked the government. Were our Supreme court justices the originalists they claim to be they would recognize the dangers of partisanship clearly seen, not in the Constitution itself, which sticks to the government, but in the Federalist Papers, written by Madison and Hamilton, primary authors of our Constitution. Were our justices really originalist they would see both the value of diversity and the problems associated with dominance—such as silencing your opponent with gerrymandering.

Something more radical is needed, and for that we turn to Jesus. Yes, that Jesus.

THE WILDERNESS RULES

No better example exists for how to deal with abusive power of any kind than Jesus' rebuke to the devil after his 40-day wilderness fast:

1. "You're hungry!" the devil tempted. "Use your power to make bread from stones."
2. "You are weak, and you have nothing. Worship me and I will give you all the wealth and power the world can offer."
3. "You are all alone. Call your angels to protect you as you jump from a pinnacle of the temple, then all who see your feat will bow down."

From these three temptations and Jesus's immediate refusals to abuse his power, we get what we call the Wilderness Rules. One's power should never be:

1. Used to satisfy a personal appetite.
2. Sold or used for personal enrichment.
3. Used to gain power over others—political, economic, or ecclesiastical.

We see in Jesus's example, plus the concept of asabiyya, the Confucian rules, and the social contract, that the proper use of power is to serve others, protect them from threats as much as possible, and help them along the path of strength and health. More than the egocentric quest for power that characterizes most of human history, the proper use of power is its combination with love, as Reverend King posited, to establish the justice that makes the field safe for all to play. That's how we build a strong society while making sure that the warp doesn't overrule the woof. It is not at all different from the advice to our confused young men today about what it means to be a man: protect others—make the playing field safe for everyone.

We would like to see the Wilderness Rules added to the Oath of Office at all levels of government. Post them in our boardrooms, too, and all other places where power is wielded, and perhaps post some wise grandmothers to watch over what goes on in those halls of power. The Wilderness Rules and the Confucian Mandate of Heaven guide the people in their choice of leaders, but rather than overthrow their government with a revolution or insurrection, it's done in a more peaceful and evolutionary way with our version of quorum sensing—voting.

Would the Rules work? There will always be ways to get around them, but they would very likely help our attorneys and investigative journalists make Martin Luther King's arc of the moral universe a bit smaller by advancing our progress toward justice.

ANALYSIS VS. EMERGENCE

Analysis is the foundation of the scientific method that took shape in the post-Newtonian world as we better understood the laws of motion. We thought we could fix everything by taking it apart, repairing or replacing the faulty parts, and putting it back together. This works well when it comes to our machines and even sometimes accidentally in our complex ecosystems. It has even been applied to our fundamental biology. Jacques Monod, a Nobel laureate for his work on how our cells work, famously said: "The cell is a machine; the animal is a machine; man is a machine."[30]

With apologies to Monod, analysis works well when systems are linear, one part connected to another in a chain. And even in the case of mixed elements, like a Rube Goldberg machine, it's still linear and easy to figure out. But in complex systems this is never the case. Networks replace linear connections, and they don't act like machines. We prefer the simpler way of analysis because those systems are easier to work with. Even when we bring computer modeling to bear on the complexity of networked systems, there are always connections left out which we do not understand. Our modeling programs remain linear, they just have many branches.

Emergence is a game-changer. It is the bridge to innovative disruption, and we have examples in both the mechanical and natural worlds:

- Deep Blue—IBM's chess-playing computer that learned to play chess on its own—is seen as a counterexample of mechanical emergence. The computer software taught itself novel approaches to the game and subsequently beat chess masters. It shows how a machine can learn something new by repetitive and recursive linear processes, but the learning is not emergent. Recursive programming is how linear programs handle webs, or networks, but they have a limit. In webs, each branch or strand needs many recursive processes, and keeping track of them quickly grows unwieldy. In the burgeoning field of artificial intelligence the branches become complex, with many internal branches requiring massive computer space. Proponents claim that some of the AI results are emergent. If that is borne out in further looking it is a massive signal for the need to regulate its development—AI is Gyges ring for the self-interested.

- In Yellowstone, nature taught us a fascinating lesson in emergence when trout in the streams flourished after wolves were reintroduced to the park, setting off an unpredictable sequence of changes. When the wolves returned, the elk that used to forage near the streams where vegetation grew more abundantly moved their foraging to the fields, where they could see danger coming. Consequently, the vegetation near the streams grew denser, providing more shade, which lowered the temperature of the water in the streams. Cooler water meant more trout and happier fishermen.

Emergence is more than simple mechanics, it is a complex interplay of many factors, closer to what Albert Einstein called "mental play." Emergence is like working a jigsaw puzzle in one's mind and seeing in flash how the pieces fit together. For Einstein, such mental play led to insights and intuitions that inspired him to formulate a revolutionary new physics.

Sometimes it's accidental. When I used xylitol in a nasal spray in a patient with asthma and asthma went away, it was emergent; I had no idea why, and my only rationale was that I knew asthma seems to be triggered in the upper airway. I was playing. But after the recognition of emergence comes the task of finding out how and why—to see if the pathway is useful in other places.

Children are the archetype of complex adaptive systems. I think that is what Jesus was looking at when he used a child as an example of what heaven is like. No other creature on earth adapts into so many different physical, social, and familial environments as a child. We can learn much by just watching them. Play is what kids do, and it's simplicity at its finest. It is repetitive, and it is active learning, with 70-80% learning retention, far higher than the alternative that dominates most school systems. Play leads to emergence, and children gain understanding from their play. The "ah ha" moments show on their faces when they gain an understanding through their play, and their parents and teachers love it. It is the state of mind that leads to emergence, so we need to cultivate it across our lands, from our preschools to our retirement communities. Play is how we gain this wonderful way of learning. We naturally utilize it all day and night as children, until the moment we walk through those school doors and into the domain of didactic learning and its 20% to 30% learning retention.

Emergence happens in evolution when speciation occurs, and reproduction is constrained to within the species. The reasons are not clear, but a different fitness landscape is one factor. Then there are the massive emergences following endosymbiosis that can change all life on this planet. Long, long ago a bacterium learned how to use sunlight to make sugars. It shared that ability by dividing, then one of these decided to play with a larger cell. They joined together, and what emerged was the world of plants, where all species share this primitive organism that we now call a chloroplast. Endosymbiosis is this joining together to make something new. It is a stellar example of the power of woof action in the sacrifice of one's individuality for the creation of something new. And the same endosymbiosis happened in the creation of the mitochondria that power all animal cells by making energy from the plants' sugars.

Mental play and mechanics are not big enough to understand emergence. The ideas that emerge like this come from the synthesis of the human mind, or even sometimes from our inner gods and goddesses. The 20th century Indian mathematician Srinivasa Ramanujan has been called a magical genius. A normal genius can explain the connections and reasons for his emergent idea. A great genius needs a special audience to understand what they are talking about. A magical genius can't begin to explain his insights. Srinivasa claimed that his astounding mathematical insights came to him from the Hindu goddess Namagiri in his dreams. Early on, many of his theorems were thought to be erroneous, but with time the overwhelming majority of them have been verified. Such insights are at the far end of emergence. They are spontaneous and seem to come from a level of the mind beyond ordinary consciousness. Although they seemingly come and go of their own volition, such emergence can be fostered and promoted. We can tap the inner genius—science understands the mechanisms of this phenomenon.[31] And if science can do it, there's reason to believe we can do it for the benefit of our society. Emergence is an inborn capacity to make big leaps.

The Skunk Works division of Lockheed Martin is famous for its 'big leap ahead' advances such as stealth technology, and looking behind the scenes one sees an organization that fosters emergence. Peer behind the scenes at Sante Fe Institute and you find a similar environment where bright, talented people thrive. Same goes for Cambridge's Cavendish Laboratories. In the obituary written by Anthony Tucker for the Lab's former director, Max Perutz, is a lesson on how to create the conditions that foster emergence:[32]

Impishly, whenever he was asked whether there are simple guidelines along which to organize research so that it will be highly creative, [Perutz] would say: no politics, no committees, no reports, no referees, no interviews; just gifted, highly motivated people picked by a few men of good judgment.

We hope Max would include women of good judgment, too.

The environment Perutz created epitomizes the safety needed for creative play; such play is not possible when threats are perceived. They also enjoy the *sense of coherence* that Aaron Antonovsky identified as common in healthy people. Control, understanding, and meaning are the hallmarks of coherence. The sense of *control* allows them to play with their toys, to be novel, to push the boundaries and explore new frontiers. Their play leads to *understanding*, a level of comprehension that leads to integration and the cross-pollination of sharing with others. And doing that increases *meaning.* It all leads to the emergence of novelty, and further to innovative disruption.

Coherence and emergence are the pillars of this book. All its suggestions are to further build up coherence and emergence and the healthy systems they foster. They are the supporting structures found in generative cultures, the ones Socrates encouraged us to copy and the ones we want to build, those "oriented on what works, where potentially damaging information is welcomed and distributed to the right people to act on."[33]

The American Academy of Arts and Sciences commissioned a study on the "Practice of Democratic Citizenship," completed in 2020. Based on historical information combined with listening sessions all over the country, their report, *Our Common Purpose,* with its suggestions based mostly on their community findings, arrived at remarkably similar suggestions.[34]

The elements of healthy people and a healthy society are not hidden away in laboratories and think tanks. They are fairly easy to promote in living and adapting organisms, be it people, communities, societies, or nations. But in every system there are impediments to the sort of playfulness behind emergence and coherence. There is no play in a fearful environment; play only happens when a person is in control and not threatened. Play is a sign of a healthy system. Danger and threat are unhealthy; they stifle play, and consequently emergence and coherence, too.

Emergence is common in children, and it's no wonder—play comes naturally to them; it's how they learn. Every teacher and parent recognizes when something clicks in the child's mind. I saw it when our two-year old granddaughter visited our home during the summer and played naked in a water-filled tub in the backyard. A look crossed her face, and I had a hunch she was pooping. I asked her if she was pooping, and something clicked—it showed on her face. Something about her freedom to play and the novelty of the moment made a connection in her mind. As her mother later reported to us, it completed her potty training.

The scientists, researchers, and others fortunate enough to be allowed to play with their work are using the pathways we all develop before institutionalized learning whips it out of us. As children, we learn by playing with objects in our environment, and learn more when those objects are familiar. My little granddaughter learned a lesson in potty training through her body that day. At that age we freely share what we learn, cross-pollinating our new understanding with others. It is healthy and begins during childhood, but only in safe, controlled environments like grandpa's backyard tub.

We can make our adult world safe and controlled, too, not just in leading-edge institutions but across society, if we first debunk the myth that we must live under the law of the jungle where self-interest and self-survival reign.

The novelty which follows emergent understanding is a driving force behind economic growth and innovations of all kinds. It's like the *invisible hand* that guides our economy, as proposed by economist Adam Smith. Smith saw this force of progress as an emergent property of a moral-based marketplace—one where the seller is equally concerned with the well-being of the buyer as his own, and the transaction is win-win. And *morals* are important because the underlying premise of *An Inquiry into the Nature and Causes of the Wealth of Nations*, where he first proposed his idea of the invisible hand guiding the marketplace, is found in his earlier work, *The Theory of Moral Sentiments.* In terms of the warp and woof, markets work best when sellers have a woof interest in their community—when their deals are win-win—rather than a warp interest solely in their personal financial condition—the win-lose option.

The world now seems headed in the win-win direction; it's what Klaus Schwab, the head of the World Economic Forum, describes as the Great Reset. The rhetoric is lofty and encouraging to hear from one of the world's most influential organizations, and in the US the Businessmen's Roundtable, made up of the leaders of major companies, has followed that lead by changing their focus from the primary neoliberal one of shareholder profits coming first, to seeing corporate responsibility as including the well-being of their communities, their workers, and their customers, as well as their shareholders.

Emergent ideas are not always beneficial, and nothing demonstrates that as well as splitting atoms. The concept arose after the instability of heavy atoms was theorized by Einstein and confirmed by English and Irish researchers. When the numbers of splitting atoms can be controlled, we can use the heat generated to make power. But there are always those who want more, and in the middle of WWII it was feared that Germany, with Werner Heisenberg, a German who knew the physics behind the process, was building a bomb. Fear, and its lizard brain responses—in this case existential—led to the Manhattan project and our bomb. And that led to an arms race where each side made enough nuclear bombs to obliterate the world.

The same sort of pro vs. con arguments can be made about the internet. The properties of silicon crystals were there just waiting to be discovered. They are not the real story here. The story is the discovery of those properties and the emergent understanding of how they could be used to contain information. On the one hand, the applications have led to a great expansion of knowledge and the easy sharing of it online. On the other hand, the profits are found elsewhere. The internet provided a simple means of collecting personal data, analyzing that data, and using it for directed advertising and political messaging (as done by Cambridge Analytica), and doing it surreptitiously. It also led to the rules for optimizing the profits, which impacts us all—mostly unconsciously.

A small group of Google programmers wrote about how their YouTube algorithm is based on deep understanding of human thinking patterns.[35] And it's not just YouTube; Meta (Facebook), Fox News, and what's left of Twitter (now called X) all put it to use. Viewer attention increases YouTube profits, so the folks calling the shots created a challenge for their employees to increase viewing time up to a billion hours *per day*. Analysis didn't work, so they looked at what did work—they played. In October 2016, they reached the goal, and the formula that emerged from their play was: *outrage equals attention, and attention equals profits*. Outrage triggers fear and our alert response; it gives us something to fight against, and it is most often driven by primitive instincts of our lizard brains—it's not conscious. Our advertisers, news outlets and social media rely on this formula to gain and hold our attention, and it locks us into survival-oriented thinking that shuts down cognitive thinking. This is not to say that there is nothing good on or about YouTube. The variety and helpfulness is there and individuals choose what to watch, but the corporate goal of all social media is profit, so there are always attractive baits to lure one on.[36] By design, it is meant to activate viewers' unconscious fears and limit their options for action. Those rules are now the pillars of the fitness landscape for social media.

D. Graham Burnett, the Princeton historian of science talks about the similarity of this process with fracking.[37] Fracking is how we get residual oil out of the ground. The only way to do this is to pump down in there high pressure, high volume detergent, which forces up to the surface this kind of slurry, mixture of natural gas, crude oil, leftover detergent, and juice and nasty stuff, which you then separate out, and you get your monetizable crude.

This is a precise analogy to what's happening to us in our contemporary attention economy. We have a [very profitable] industry, which, to get the money value of our attention out of us, is continuously pumping into our faces high-pressure, high-value detergent in the form of social media and non-stop content that holds us on our devices. And that pumping brings to the surface that spume, that foam of our attention, which can be aggregated and sold off to the highest bidder.

Money seems to have replaced words in much of our communication.

The other face of emergence is in the world of biology, where it is even more common. The absence of money in nature allows the fitness landscape to be about survival. But survival in nature, as we have seen, is dual just like our warp and woof; it can be competitive—virulent—or commensal—cooperative. Earlier, we touched on a prime example found in dental research with xylitol that resulted in bacteria building plaque on our teeth that actually prevents tooth decay. That was a very beneficial emergent process. There are lots of other bacteria living in us that are just as much a part of our defenses as the ones on our teeth which have adapted for our benefit. Like the trout in Yellowstone that thrived in the cooler water, we can frame our fitness landscape to guide us, both personally and as a nation, to improved health.

Sometimes, emergent mutations feed new adaptations. Early human communities communicated with sounds. The San people of southern Africa are the oldest indigenous group we know of, and they still use clicking sounds in their speech. This primitive speech became part of the fitness landscape for further mutations, and further success led to the emergence of language. Language led to the emergence of cultural memories and storytelling, which led to not only extended relationships but also helped to build stronger limbic systems where those relationships are remembered and the personal smells that lead to intimacy are recognized.[38, 39,40] Then we developed writing systems that use words, and the fitness landscape adjusted to include rational thinking about how to put those words together to convey a meaningful message.[41] This in turn led to the emergence of *genesis* stories, and religion, and science; and science led to more advanced thinking technology, but the connection and the role of the fitness landscape in this chain of adaptations is seldom mentioned.

We began with basic sound and built new, emergent adaptations step by step all the way up to a formalized system for teaching everyone how to think scientifically and thereby gain greater understanding of the world and life itself. And all along the way the success of mutations was guided by a fitness landscape that also grew in complexity along with the agents of change.

It is likely that the inbreeding we use today in animal husbandry to enhance desirable characteristics played a natural role in our prehistorical, small tribal units, where it worked similarly to enhance a variety of novel characteristics. None could be predicted in advance, and, as with all mutations, most of them wound up in the garbage. But proliferation followed for the ones that fit the landscape, and once we see and understand an emergent property, we can use it. That is what science does in the lab and entrepreneurs do in the business world, and it is what we all should be doing with history if we don't want to endlessly repeat our mistakes!

That is one reason why the study of history is so important—it shows how people adapt. When it is not written by the winners, it is the best source we have for what has worked. It gives one the ability to foresee and understand our adaptations in history, and to form our political and social plans based on what has worked before. In it we can see what emerges; it's what political philosopher and noted student of autocracy, Hannah Arendt, was talking about when she said, "Beginning, before it becomes a historical event, is the supreme capacity of man; politically, it is identical with man's freedom."[42]

Understanding how and why we choose a path of action is true freedom. If our decision-making is cognitive rather than fear-based, it allows us to observe the spur-of-the-moment, unconscious, and mostly tactical thinking which leads us astray. When the fitness landscape is about profits we make virulence, or self-interest, the better choice. But just as with the world of nature there are two paths: virulence or commensalism; self-interest or cooperation. The question is, how do we open the door to cooperation wider? Doing that is the beginning, before the historical fact, is looking for what is emerging—and it is the basis of our freedom.

Outrage and fear are the fitness landscape of our current model of social media and much of our news because profits define what works. But fear puts one in their lizard brain, where cooperation is anathema. Needless to say, both sides of our political spectrum use fear tactics against their opponents, and I suggest such use is a measuring stick to determine who is unfit to serve the people. Resorting to fear tactics makes one unworthy because it eliminates cognitive thinking. It's one thing when a threat is aimed at ways of thinking. Cognitive threats leave room to argue, and argument in this sense is healthy—it's arguing to learn. We need only look at the vigorous debate between various individuals and factions around the time of the founding of our republic to see the difference between that sort of argument and today's threats aimed at egos and belief systems. Existential threats trigger the primal brain to act up, and the cortex, the higher brain, to shut down, and ego threats do the same thing.

Building a healthy nation means building healthy communities, because they are the foundation of our nation, as de Tocqueville and many others have pointed out. In seeking solutions, we can look to the billions of years of experience of the microbial world where diverse microbial communities are the norm; but creating them is complicated. Researchers from Yale looked at microbial communities and found they are not unlike ours in their diversity. But in order to study them, they took them apart, the classic "dissect under a microscope" approach of all analytical studies. But interestingly, when those researchers tried to put everything back together the way it was, mixing the various microbial colonies together, they encountered the microbial version of red-lining, known as "competitive exclusion," which is essentially what Kevin Phillips found in the ethnic boroughs of New York. The "melting pot" butted up against reality, and the researchers concluded that such communities are emergent; they are not amenable to analysis.[43] Were I in that lab I would check to see if those removed from the colony and kept as a separate species lost their glycan coats in the process so that they lost the ability to communicate with the colony. It suggests that policies that force integration are doomed to failure. And that goes for forcing any kind of social change.

The opposite can also be found. Lee Kwan Yew, the former Prime Minister of Singapore, also faced ethnic challenges among the dominant Malay, the prosperous Chinese, and the minority Indians. He dealt with it, not by legislation, but by altering the landscape; he established a housing policy in city-built apartment complexes that mandated occupancy proportional to that of the population. It resulted in less ethnic division. The people of the various ethnicities began thinking of themselves as Singaporeans, and intermarrying made it real. Lee's idea could have come from the US military seventeen years earlier with its Presidential integration in 1948, with the same results as far as integration and intermarriage. While there was lots of resistance, an autocrat was in charge—the military was his child.

To make America healthy again, we can begin by creating environments that bring out the best in people. Environments where we can freely generate creative solutions to their problems. Environments free of fear and coercion. We can find ways of reaching across boundaries and dividing lines and teaching that the cooperative pathway is not only better in the long run, it's healthier, too. We will not analyze our way to the answers to these difficult problems. The answers emerge organically when we create the right environment.

COUNTERWILL

First described by psychologist Otto Rank, one of Sigmund Freud's colleagues, and picked up later by psychologist Gordon Neufeld in his work with children, counterwill is our instinct to resist coercion and outside control. Any top-down control generates counterwill, be it in children or society. We can see it affecting the people in our body politic who fear becoming minorities in a rapidly diversifying society; the people who think government regulations steal their ability to act freely; and the people watching helplessly as powerful neighbors and large corporations destroy their communities. We can see it in the blowback from *Brown v. Board of Education,* the Supreme Court decision that integrated our schools, only to have them equally segregated seventy years later by a growing population of private schools. People lack control, *t*hey feel coerced, and as a result they rebel, whether openly or subversively. That decision directly affected everyone in the United States. It came from above, was seen as intrusive, and built counterwill. Discussions aimed at reaching a consensual decision would not likely have worked. But what if the fitness landscape included a federal grant for integrating a school district. It may have taken longer but the end result would be better than what we have today.

Either way, counterwill is normal and mostly healthy for society. It's even unhealthy to *not* have it in cases where it is needed. Counterwill gave birth to our nation, as the colonists revolted against the coercive control of the British. Counterwill is needed to balance society.

But these days, counterwill has been hijacked by many using the ease of inducing outrage in our online speech. The flood of information available on the Internet easily facilitates the conspiracy minded to find collusion in coincidence and causation in correlation, both of which are errors of judgment without more supporting data. The printed outrages also escape any liability or verification by being covered by the free speech granted in the First Amendment.

The extent and nature of current counterwill is demonstrated in the explosion of online and public threats to New York County District Attorney Alvin Bragg after Donald Trump announced that he was going to be arrested by him. Many of them were death threats. Such counterwill shows that it extends to the tribe of those being threatened even though it does not affect them. They are more indicative of the blind flocking behavior seen in the Nazi treatment of Jews.

In much the same way, counterwill is behind much of the polarization of our society. People pushed to lizard brain thinking by persistent threats tend to form flocks, or schools, as birds and fish do when predators are nearby. People form tribes, at least that's what many call them. It's difficult to accept that usage if we listen to what Kondiaronk told the Baron de Lahontan, since the chief had no direct power to persuade tribal members; only after long deliberation was a choice of action determined. I would use the term mob-like rather than tribal to describe the actions of those caught up in persistent midbrain thinking. And if they have a leader who maintains their allegiance, the group becomes mob-like in nature. To be beneficial, groupthink must maintain the cognitive thinking of the individuals, and focus on arguing to learn rather than arguing to win.

The best historical example took place in Germany in 1933, when Hitler created an enemy: the Jews and the Communists (frequently conflated). In much the same way, immigrants, Muslims, and the persecutors of Trump are the enemies created by our true-believers in the US. The violence committed by both the Nazi Brownshirts and American right-wing militias are aimed at their so-called enemies. Savvy propagandists tap into the counterwill of disaffected elements of a society and direct it for political gain.[44] We sensed that with the Russian involvement in the 2016 presidential election. Observers see it up close in the 2024.[45]

The study of counterwill began with looking at it in children, so it's fitting that we look there for a means of dealing with it. According to the American Academy of Pediatrics (AAP), the best tool for guiding a child's adaptation is not corporal or verbal punishment; it's to show them that the desired behavior is in their best interest. It's a process of mediation to reach a consensual decision—it's not based on power.[46] The use of fairy tales or Aesop's Fables also accomplishes this goal by teaching and imparting knowledge through story.

The authors at AAP did not mention counterwill but should have since it underlies their whole program. Empowerment through offering choice is nonthreatening and continues to foster a safe environment where children can play and learn. It puts the parent in the role of teacher rather than dictator. And the kicker is it works with any person or adaptive system, from bacterial biofilms to nation-states. There's tremendous potential for applying these insights to solving our problems instead of creating more of them.

Understanding counterwill is a master password for cracking the code that's programming us as individuals and as societies to rebel rather than cooperate. Not only can we increase the health of the body politic, but we can also break the grip that threats have on our thinking. As a society, we are traumatized; the constant threats to our egos from advertisers, who show us what we need to have in order to fit, and political fundraisers creating fear of the opposition, trigger the same type of response as do the existential threats behind PTSD in the military, and the sooner we diagnose it, the sooner we can treat it. PTSD is not just a problem for soldiers who've been through combat; the fear we all feel leads to a society full of traumatized people who can't break out of the cycle.

The result of resolving counterwill by discussing and recommending the best path forward—at all levels—is the ability to structure together a fitness landscape that aids the adaptation. One of the best ways to show that is found in the Prisoner's Dilemma.

THE PRISONER'S DILEMMA

Survive on your own, or survive through cooperation—which is better? These are the twin paths of evolution, which we call the warp and the woof, and they can be tested through a game known as the Prisoner's Dilemma. Darwin would love this game. He was fascinated with what makes some civilizations survive and thrive and others collapse and disappear, and the Prisoner's Dilemma provides the evidence that answers the question.

The Prisoner's Dilemma is a common game in psychological

research. A couple is caught in a crime. As they are separately interrogated they and presented with the choice of ratting out their partner or not. If they rat—the word used is "defect"—then they can get a better deal and the erstwhile partner gets penalized. If the prisoner does not defect but instead *cooperates* with his partner by staying mum, then their collective fate is likely to be less severe because there is less information to use against them. If they both defect, then no one wins. This game has been modified to work in other situations with rewards to fit: single defectors get $5, and their partners lose $3; mutual cooperators get $3 each; and mutual defectors get nothing. The players make their choices not knowing what the other one decided.

So, you have a situation where choices can lead to all or nothing (win-lose), nothing-nothing (lose-lose), or a guaranteed something for both players (win-win). Computerized versions of the game include the added complexity of social interactions trying to modify your partner's future choices. Run the game enough times and the long-term results provide the kind of information Darwin needed to understand the rise and fall of civilization. Cooperative societies rise because cooperation leads to higher fitness, which in a commodified society like ours means more money. The Social Darwinist all-or-nothing (win-lose) competition leads to lower fitness and health and actually less money to go around. Players in society who only look out for number-one in the perverted Social Darwinist sense weaken the fabric of society.

The defectors gain an advantage because they are more willing to use others to get ahead, and they can find partners who see them as more powerful and willing to follow. They "win" at the expense of the cooperators.[47] It's the same situation as that described earlier about self-interest versus altruism. Selling your naïve partner on staying mum while you defect is a win for the self-interested but a loss for the group.

With this information, Darwin could show how natural selection also applies to civilizations—the pathway is just more complex. It makes the fallacy of Social Darwinism clear. Empathy, not competitive self-interest, wins. But he was never able to bridge that gap, leaving the door open for others to pervert his ideas to justify defecting, competition, inequality, and caste. The defectors' "all take and no give" strategy gives them a short-term advantage, but their exploitation means that everyone loses in the long run because the health of the collective affects the health of the individual and vice-versa. That is the Prisoner's Dilemma.

Another argument for this point of view comes from anthropologist Brian Hare and writer Vanessa Woods in *Survival of the Friendliest.*[48] They looked at the social changes in dogs, bonobos, and humans as they adapted to their environmental niches over a span of thousands of years. They started with foxes, specifically the *Siberian fox experiment*. It began 1959 when geneticist Dimitri Belyaev selected foxes for inbreeding that showed less fear of humans. Over subsequent generations, the foxes increased their social intelligence. Their ears grew floppy, their heads smaller, and their tails curlier—they became "lap foxes." The same thing changed wolves into dogs as they adapted to human interaction through a symbiotic relationship of feasting on the humans' food leftovers.

Bonobos adapted to a non-threatening environment where food was plentiful by moving toward a noncompetitive female-dominant society. The competitive, defector-like males are pulled back into a cooperative society by female sharing, including the sharing of sexual favors.[49] When there's enough to go around for everyone and no scarcity, people cooperate. Animals do, too.

But introduce scarcity—even the thought of scarcity, as in the Great Replacement threat—and the competition kicks in, which means that some win and some lose. In societies of high complexity like ours, where the warp of self-interest has been the dominant paradigm for the last fifty years, the result is an abundance of defectors with more money and power, and their naïve financial supporters, the losers with less of it. Society becomes less fit in evolutionary terms.

The introduction of religion provided the glue that the woof needed for society to advance, and it is an example of natural selection because groups and societies that organized around a common religion were more likely to survive. "For, it was the push for capacity for more sociality and group formation among hominins over millions of years of evolution that made religion part of all human societies."[50] Unfortunately, though, the warp of ecumenical power is just as corrupting as political power, and the fracturing of religion into various tribes has incorporated ego identification and social pressures so that religious tribes have evolved more on the defector warp path of survival than the cooperative woof path.

All religions maintain a fundamental interest in the value of *the other*: the stranger, the traveler, those in need. Even self-centered neoliberalism has fostered a prosperity-focused religious movement—more wealth enables more trickle-down charity. A question that remains unanswered is whether a return to the cooperative paradigm that our religions started with would push society toward more community orientation. The answer to the question lies in figuring out a solution to scarcity.

The Prisoner's Dilemma offers a lesson to get us started in that direction by choosing the right political leaders. Many people enter politics because it enhances their ability to defect, to gain power and be able to profit from deal-making and privileged information. On the other side are those people motivated by a genuine desire to serve. How do we tell the difference? We could run them through the Prisoner's Dilemma game to get an idea of whether they are the "I know better than you" type, or the "nothing about us without us" type. But time is the true test—a person's true character emerges over time. Or we could ask their grandmothers what they think!

The bottom line learned from the Prisoner's Dilemma is that the cooperators in this dance of evolution lead their society to greater evolutionary fitness. The defectors harm everyone in the long run, including themselves. This realization leads us to look for why we continue to make choices that lead us down a path of less evolutionary fitness, and for that answer we turn to how the brain works.

SYSTEM 1 AND SYSTEM 2: THE ELEPHANT AND THE RIDER

Nature has many defense mechanisms. Among the better-known are the bitter alkaloids acacia trees send out to foraging giraffes, and the use of quorum sensing by bacteria to signal each other. But while crises increase the rate of mutation across the board, change by natural selection is still a slow process. Animals with nervous systems have developed a much faster system. To see it in action, put your hand on something hot and see how fast your nervous system tells you to pull it away. For good reason, natural selection has made burn signals travel extremely fast, but there's another type of damage that works slowly, and it may take months or years to get the message. It's the damage caused by trauma, and our society is experiencing a full-blown epidemic of it.

To understand trauma and its effects, we begin with how signals are carried to the brain and processed. The damage caused by trauma is like the signals from bruising or penetrating injuries that may not be noticed until minutes after the fact, except with other forms of trauma, like sexual abuse of a child, it may take months or years to get the message. The brain also has two response systems, one slow and deliberate and the other a flash in the pan, and our understanding of how they work provides a pathway to healing ourselves and our nation. One response system—System 1—activates in the blink of an eye because it bypasses the cognitive brain to produce reflex-like action. It's tantamount to the alert stress response discussed earlier in Chapter Three and elsewhere. Therapist Resmaa Menakem calls it our "lizard brain" and I like the term too because it paints a vivid picture of its evolutionary origins, and it makes us more aware of its limited options.[51] Lizards and reptiles in general look out for number-one and will battle each other to the death for resources and supremacy, so when we look for what brings out this behavior in people, look no further than the lizard brain.

Once thought of as a simple and straightforward mechanism for triggering fight-or-flight response, the integrated stress response is more complex. It triggers our bodies to fight or flee, but it also influences body development: as noted earlier, our muscles get bigger and our brains get smaller.[52] This curious fact was confirmed by a study looking at the connections between the brain and the heart. As the structures in the primitive brain get larger from sending out hormones and messages related to danger, so does the heart muscle get bigger to send blood to the body's muscles.[53] It's an evolutionary gift that helps us escape danger. And another curious finding is that ego threats trigger our instinctive survival responses as much as existential threats do. Unfortunately, these cellular controls are all geared to enhance survival—the warp—at the expense of cortical development and one's health—the woof.[54]

Many researchers agree with the idea that the health disparities like higher rates of chronic disease and premature death seen in our ethnically Black population result from underlying racial prejudice. It's not just about genetics; social elements of the environment, mostly threats, influence health in these same ways. Genetics may play some role in passing on traits that create health disparities, but look deeper and the stress response bears some culpability; specifically, the cascade of effects it triggers physiologically and psychologically.

One of the best examples of this is the mysterious drop in the mortality rate of Black babies in Madison, Wisconsin, from 19.4 per thousand between 1990 to 2001, down to 6.4 per thousand between 2002 to 2007. Doctors and healthcare specialists analyzed this result down to 'the chemicals in the paint' and could find no scientific or medical cause. Analysis doesn't work in complex systems. This drop correlates with the presence of a clinic in Madison that catered to the Black community. It was called a Harambee—a Swahili word meaning "working together." The Harambee brought midwives together with pregnant women in the community, and from there the number tells the story of the good it did. While correlation is not causation, every mammal needs a safe place to deliver and care for their offspring, and when it is not available some mammals will even eat their offspring. The Harambee provided it.

A Veteran's Administration study found the same thing when looking at cardiac outcomes: "In a setting where differences in access [to health care] are minimized, so are racial differences in functional status outcomes."[55]

When we are safe and thinking clearly, we can gain the objectivity to think through and respond to problems, but the responses affecting our genes do their work without our awareness. The *perception of a threat* kicks the body into high gear. It shunts blood from the GI tract and other nonessential organs to the muscles and the heart so that a person can outrun, outmaneuver, and escape or neutralize the threat. Freezing is the other option if fighting or fleeing are not possible, but it's not right to say it's an option—we don't choose it, it's instinctive, and it works when there's no other hope for survival. For example, animals taken down by large predators often freeze and appear dead until an opportunity arises to escape. Now correlate that response with children confronted by environments of constant physical and psychological threat—they often respond similarly by withdrawing into themselves. The evolutionary path from reptile to human can clearly be seen, and so can the reason for why so many people are unable to function optimally in society.

If threats keep us from cognitive functioning, and our world is permeated with threats, how do we apply this insight to society to make it healthy? The answer is to create the conditions that move us away from stress responses, and to do that we begin by eliminating as much stress as possible, and also by teaching strategies for dealing with it when it's unavoidable.

For when it's unavoidable, we have examples and strategies offered by people like Resmaa Menakem in his book *My Grandmother's Hands*, and by organizations like the Arbinger Institute and their book *The Anatomy of Peace*. It tells the story of two young, like-minded men who met at school. One's father was killed by Palestinians in the Intifada, and the other's father was killed by the Israeli army in the West Bank. Each had a load of resentment, fear of the other, and hate. But they were united in their desire to find a way out, and it brought them together by honoring every person, helping make a safe place in their lives, and finding the best path forward together. It's what the Haudenosaunee do in their longhouse discussions.

Like microbes, stress is everywhere in modern society. It's inescapable, especially in social environments of scarcity and dog-eat-dog competition. And like an animal caught by a predator, when we can't fight or flee, our instinctive response is to drop out, freeze, or even die—figuratively or literally. The commensal approach, steeped in empathy, prompts us to change the environmental conditions—the fitness landscape that determines the success or failure of a novelty—for the benefit of everyone. We can make evolution conscious.

That's what both Daniel Kahneman and Jonathan Haidt seem to be aiming at in their popular books on the subjects of survival and healthy pathways in our brains, showing how they work and just how powerful and prevalent they are, but neither author delves into its evolutionary origins nor acknowledges the limitations of survival thinking.[56,57] Kahneman, a psychologist and economist, divides our thought processes into "System 1" and "System 2." System 1 is the instinctual fight-or-flight response that dominates our unconscious thinking. He calls it "fast thinking" because it is reflexive. System 2 is slower and more cognitive; it's the healthy pathway involving the frontal and prefrontal cortex, the parts of our brains that make us *Homo sapiens* and allow for strategic thinking, but that are shut down when fast thinking is in control.

Jonathan Haidt, a social psychologist, uses the metaphor of

the elephant (the System 1 instinctual *and powerful* pathway) and a rider on the elephant (the System 2 logical and reasoning pathway, less powerful but far-seeing and strategic). The rider is the cortical brain that sees problems ahead, before they register on the elephant, and may resolve them before the elephant's survival reflexes kick in. Once the elephant is in danger-mode, it's much more difficult to steer in a better direction. The rider in this metaphor represents the superior evolutionary path of cortical thinking that enhances survival and health, and the key insight is that the rider must be able to see ahead and avert danger before it materializes—he needs to be a student of history.

Kahneman and Haidt both focus on the duality seen in the midbrain, the fast-thinking part, and the slower reasoning of the rider, the cortex. Left out is the limbic brain, the part dealing with our relationships. That's the part that is obliquely addressed when our leaders dehumanize their enemies by labeling them vermin or murderers. In Haidt's book titled *The Righteous* Mind, he points out that we need those labels because we can't justify doing what we intend to do to these people if they are humans; they need to be less; they need to be *other*—or they need to be guilty. The lynchings of Black men in America a century ago was justified by the stories of their abuse of white women. Justification is by faith, as the Apostle Paul told the Romans; those participating believed they were witnessing justice done. They felt justified. Such actions are easy to rationalize. So, when people join that faithful flock by the action of baptism, or buying a ticket to the rally, or other rites of passage, they are sanctified as members of the group. And when they contribute by giving their blood, tithes, or whatever is most precious to them, they find the sense of safety and security that we all desire. Then the Thomas theorem takes effect: Situations defined as real become real in their consequences. Sociologists William and Dorothy Thomas devised this theorem around the time that rampant lynchings were being questioned; one cannot help but wonder if there is a connection.

The woof in our societal tapestry is the cortical thinking of System 2. It's the rider on the elephant that sees ahead and thinks strategically about how to avoid threats so that the System 1 brain can relax. We can thank System 2 for the higher forms of thinking that rise above the perception of threat and survival-only priorities. The System 2 pathway in the brain gives us creative problem-solving, strategy and healthy adaptations. System 2 is where we label our feelings and decide on what is just—based on facts, on what is fair to all concerned, and on the love that Dr. King said should guide our use of power.

Being the rider on the elephant requires a mind that can handle the increased complexity of thinking strategically, with far-seeing vision. The healthy pathway of evolution is one of diversity. It's cooperative. Darwin saw it as a builder of civilization. We call it the woof pathway and show its foundation in the elements discussed in this chapter, as well as other elements that add to resilience—the ability to recover from adversity—which lead to better health not just for the individual, but for the family, community, nation, and world.

RESILIENCE

Resilience is characterized by the individual assets and relational and contextual resources one has access to in order to survive.[58] Individual assets are about *control* and commitment in partnership with others that is *meaningful* enough to merit the effort.

Relational resources are about the support gained from others which adds *meaning*. Contextual resources include those of education—or *understanding* the nature of the challenge—as well as access to the many local resources available to help. These are the cornerstones of individual resilience in the larger sense, encompassing more than merely physical health.

When building resilient systems, as in ecosystems, diversity is always the first element. Everything is in relationship with everything else, and the greater the diversity, the greater the pool of common resources that build resilience. Also, diversity supplies much of the understanding and the meaning behind novel solutions that more often come from cross-pollination, and the support of friends augments one's control. Resilience is the ability to bounce back from any stressful event in our lives, and it is another way to promote a healthy woof.

In the early 1980s, family researchers produced a model showing the fundamentals of resilient and healthy families:

- They *understand* the stress and how to use the resources to deal with it.
- They have a sense of *control* over the stress.
- The *meaning* they give to the stress makes it manageable rather than overwhelming.[59]

Parallel to these family therapists, sociologist Aaron Antonovsky studied what makes healthy people and found that some are just healthier than others.[60] It led him to formulate the concept of salutogenesis—the origins of health. He found it in a *sense of coherence*, which he broke down into essentially the same elements that make resilient families: a sense of control, understanding, and meaning. It tells us specifically what makes us resilient and what resilience leads to: healthy people. His test for coherence has been validated by European physicians following his ideas.

When one looks at these findings in individuals and families, together with the warp and the woof of evolution, it's easy to get excited about the prospects for applying them to the bigger picture. These researchers discovered not only the way to healthier families and humans, but to all living systems, all the way up to our nation-states. Antonovsky's *sense of coherence* provides a number of ideas that could be used in rebuilding helpful fitness landscapes for conscious evolution. Coherence is built on control, understanding, and meaning, and these conditions can be built and encouraged; they can fit very nicely into a wise fitness landscape. They can be as simple as optimizing the defenses in our airways with a simple nasal spray.

When I presented these ideas to a conference on complexity in health care, many in the audience grasped the possibility of jumping over complexity, with all its interconnections and complications, by just focusing on building coherence—by looking at what works and what helps our defenses, both personal and social. Take any problem or issue related to personal or collective health, and the answer is probably a sense of coherence. Both coherence and resilience are fundamental to health.

Control is built by empowering the person with information and means. A sense of control is both the opposite of, and the treatment for, learned helplessness, which you'll recall is part and parcel of the divide and conquer strategy. Control means the agent, the person in the eye of the storm, is in charge and has the means of coping. *Understanding* is built with reliable information from experts and others with the right experience, whether it be a teacher, coach, minister, or wise grandparent.

Provided in a safe environment, control promotes playing with the problem—the way children and those in our play-friendly laboratories devise novel solutions. It's also comparable to the play of our immune system as it strives in the germinal centers of our lymph nodes to optimize its response to an infecting organism by creating mutations until the right one is found to counteract the infection. *Meaning* is mostly found in working with others to cope with the problem, best done with those who have experienced it.[61]

For Antonovsky, coherence is the basis of *salutogenesis.* Following the woof pathway outlined by these principles can make the nation, its citizens, and the world healthy again.

However, resilience studies carried out after the original ones in the 1980s produced a mixed bag, and the reason for it is the researchers studied control but left out understanding and meaning. One such study conducted in the Middle East with children affected by war found that building control did not help the children of fundamentalist families where God/Allah was in total control.[62] In these children, a measure of learned helplessness is built-in, and the studies needed to look at more than just one of the variables. The three elements may remind one of the Three-Body Problem in mathematics. If we can be as successful in applying TBP thinking to society and health as the brewers have been with making beer—where just three ingredients combine to produce thousands of variations—playing with these three elements should make us all a bit happier.

'Play therapists' use toys with children to help them work

through the issues they are dealing with, and therapists are told to trust the process. That's what's missing in the Middle East study. Even when external events devastate one's life, local control is possible through play in a safe environment. Resilience, salutogenesis, and health are emergent processes; they are not amenable to the analytical processes that look only at one variable.

This view is based on a sense *of control*, factual *understanding*, and the *meaning* that comes with community action and help from, and for, others. It is the bigger picture of healthy soil, the environments where humans thrive, and these elements are just as much a part of defense medicine as are physiological ones. Promoting them is very much a function of good local government. It is something that can and should be fostered by good policies at all levels of government. In a real sense it is why governments exist.

Only one of the purposes of government listed in the Preamble of the Constitution—"provide for the common defense"—has anything to do with the warp "survival of the fittest" as commonly understood. The United States has performed well in this area; we have the biggest stick in town, and use it regularly, so much so that our Defense Department should be renamed the Department of Offense. Like the medical-industrial complex, the military one just keeps getting bigger and bigger at the expense of the other functions of government. We need to look again at George Kennan's "long telegram" and realize with him that building a better society is the defensive medicine that balances the offensive focus of the MIC. And just as in health care, both offense and defense are needed. Supporting the defense means addressing the unity, justice, tranquility, general welfare, and concern for liberty that the Founding Fathers recognized and honored as being the purpose of government. It means providing a safe place for productive play, which emphasizes the value of cross-pollination within our diverse population. It means that Black and Native American lives matter as much as the white elite; and it means there should be no elite ruling class or gender.

We need to find a way to move beyond survival and follow the healthy pathway toward win-win, strategic, long-term solutions to our problems. In 1990, Elinor Ostrom pointed the way when she showed, in *Governing the Commons,* how to rescue the commons from its ever-present tragedy by empowering those locally that used it, but had no control over it—an idea that won her, a political scientist, the Nobel Prize in economics in 2009.

TRAGEDY OF THE COMMONS

An economic and social problem became apparent in 19th century England due largely to a rapid increase in population. The 'tragedy of the commons' occurs when powerful individuals and organizations overuse their community's common resources and destroy their future value for other community members. Back then, the commons were the lands rented out by the wealthy nobility to people who would work them. Today, property rights control most of the land, so the remaining commons are the air we breathe, the water we drink, the earth we live on, and all the resources shared in common.

The story of the tragedy begins at the common grazing grounds for livestock animals. The arrangement worked great as long as all the animals had enough to eat, but adding more animals led to problems like overgrazing that destroyed the resource. The winner, the one with the power to continue hogging resources, could grow and sell their livestock, and the losers couldn't.

Next, the story expands to include the commons shared by entire nations. Rapid industrialization in Great Britain destroyed its environment on a scale never before seen on Earth, but the industrialists argued that they were helping society. Claiming that more people were working, and the country was getting richer, they forgot to mention that they got the lion's share of the wealth. That was the environment in which Marx wrote *Das Kapital.* The environmental destruction caused by their factories wasn't their problem. They continued to overuse the country's resources, and society paid the bill for their profits, leading to environmental destruction and resource depletion. That is the tragedy.

Overuse destroyed the self-sustaining ability of the soil and robbed the community of its future productivity. Grazing fields withered and were no longer able to feed as many livestock animals as previous years. In our day, we see the same pattern of abuse in the shift in corporate ethos away from being responsible public entities that protect the interests of the workers, the community, and the environment, favoring instead the interests of shareholders. Profits are paramount. As a result, industrial waste and pollution are dumped into the environmental commons because it is cheaper than cleaning it up responsibly. Plus, polluters can get away with it, using their wealth to blind the eyes of regulators and politicians. Resources are hoarded and depleted with no thought for the future.

The entire planet is the commons: air, water, soil, and all life, including us. And it is all under dire threat because of exploitation. If you want the best reason for why self-interest must be balanced with collective interest, look at Ostrom's work.

Lin's research showed that cooperative action could rescue the commons from destruction.[63] Bottom-up community leadership is better for human governance, but it requires pushing control downward to the people in the community, not upward to autocrats, CEOs, and experts, who are often even the owners of the land they abuse. Control at the community level is especially important for the disenfranchised in the commons. They have *understanding* of the problems, and the *meaning* that comes from participation in the community. When understanding and meaning are present, we need only add *control* to achieve coherence. Empowered people playing as a community with the elements in their environment leads to win-win problem-solving, a fact that Elinor clearly proved.

But we are headed in the opposite direction by selling control to powerful interests outside of our communities, interests that neither meaningfully participate in nor understand local issues and problems. Or we hand the responsibility to government agencies that then exert top down control that, even when their actions are in the public's best interest, is altogether too easy to turn into counterwill. Take electric power and natural gas for example, both are increasingly under the control of multinational conglomerates. The company delivering electric power to Tucson, Arizona is located in Canada. The company delivering natural gas to Bangor, Maine is headquartered in Montana, and is a subsidiary of a company headquartered in Connecticut but incorporated in Delaware. I'd be surprised if the corporate executives making the decisions that affect Bangor could locate the city on a map, but they could tell you down to the dollar the amount of profit they make off its citizens. The same sort of removal of local control and connection is happening in countless ways in communities everywhere.

Connections of personal interest outside the community break attachment to it. Powerful people can "sell out." They are the defectors in the Prisoner's Dilemma game, and they are the number-one reason why our commons are quickly depleting, and our republic, one of the grandest experiments in governance in human history, exists only in name.

SAVING OUR REPUBLIC

In sum, the shifting balance of power in our government follows the economic powers in our society, and those with the power want to keep and increase it. They tend to be defectors, and they are leading us astray. For the past half-century, neoliberal policies have dramatically increased wealth at the top, but their gain is our loss. Time Magazine says this transfer of funds from the bottom 90% of the population to the top 1% amounts to fifty trillion dollars. More money means more power, and more power means more money. A series of Supreme Court rulings, most notably *Citizens United*, have favored the defectors in society and effectively turned the nation into a plutocracy. Voting and lobbying our government used to give the people a say in how we are governed, but the political power of wealthy donors, corporations, and special interests now drowns out our voices. Money doesn't just talk, it monopolizes the conversation, while our government turns a deaf ear to its citizens.

Citizens United allows for unlimited political spending by outside interests, even ones not in the United States, as long as it is not directly controlled by the political candidates it favors, but the rule is easily skirted with a wink and a nudge. To make matters worse, the outside interests playing such a huge role in determining who gets elected often lack the ethical standards we put on candidates, leaving us with a situation where we focus on the puppet but not on the hand controlling it. Big Money games the political system in ways that are so sophisticated, not even the experts fully grasp the complexity. We see the same sort of purposeful obfuscation through complexity happening in medicine and finance, too. It's a ploy to keep the public from understanding what's really happening.

We are not going to save our republic with more counter-will-building regulations and top-down control from experts and bureaucrats. Instead, we need to give bottom-up control to the people. Tell the experts to bug off. They only run us in circles.

We are not going to save our republic by continuing to play a winner-take-all game. The only healthy path is the one where everyone wins through cooperation and compromise.

We are not going to save our republic by reacting tactically to threats with our lizard brains instead of using our cognitive brains to look at causes and address them strategically. The healthy path forward will be found by seeing beyond the threats and over the walls that define our basins of interest.

We are not going to save our republic by continuing to hammer away at specific elements of resilience and making the body politic vulnerable to opportunistic infection. We need to strengthen our defenses by promoting a sense of coherence at all levels of society.

To save our republic, we need to protect our commons, even if it means the loss of profit for some. Our political system has never been perfect, but before the cancer of money metastasized throughout the body politic, it was at least able to respond to existential threats brought about by capitalism run amok, as we did during the Progressive Era.

Some people say that we must overrule the Supreme Court's *Citizens United* decision to have any hope of ridding us of the corrupting influence of money in politics, but I think we are long past that point. It would only take us back to where we were in 2010, and by then the nation was already run by the plutocrats. Just look at the fact that the personal net worth of members of presidential cabinets has skyrocketed by *10,000%* since the Reagan era and peaked with Trump's cabinet, which was packed with self-serving plutocrats. They are *entrenched* in the political system, and they think of the people as the enemy. They will *never* give up their positions willingly. The public senses this, and enough of it rallied behind an outsider perceived as having the power to cope with the entrenched government—to "drain the swamp"—to elect him president. But they miss the fact that his narcissism leads to the power that corrupts absolutely.

I could cite more studies and statistics and roll out experts galore, but wouldn't that just be falling into the same trap we face when we walk into a doctor's office with a serious problem and get bombarded with head-spinning terms and numbers? We wind up giving control of our health to the same experts who benefit from its absence, who get rich from illness and misfortune. The health of our nation and our world must be our responsibility, and not only the problems but the solutions must be within *everyone's* ability to know and grasp.

As a physician for the past 50 years, I've seen the best outcomes from patients who took control of their own health. I've witnessed miraculous recoveries and seen families and communities rally to support each other. The prognosis for our nation's health is not good, but harping on that fact is not good, either. The Thomas theorem tells us as much—if we think all is lost, it becomes a self-fulfilling prophecy. But I'm not saying that pretending everything is kosher will make it so. Instead, I'm saying that we know what the problems are and how to fix them, that we can fix our nation's health by following the same principles we use to fix the body's. We can end the warfare mentality and learn from the microbes that have been around on this planet since life originated. They have much to teach us, and lesson number-one is the interests of the community must come first.

I remember when Ronald Reagan campaigned on the idea of reducing government. He convinced many people that it was the best path forward. While he did not reduce government, his ideological followers, like Steve Bannon, Trump's political strategist, believe that it's best to destroy the government and let the cards fall where they may. Out of the chaos will come a *new order*, but if crisis and opportunity go hand in hand as suggested by the Chinese character for chaos, in a defector society the opportunity goes to the powerful. We could benefit from less government, but we certainly do not need to destroy it.

We need a government that functions properly and is spread locally so that it's not some distant stranger trying to control your life. It's instead a local face in your community who understands your unique challenges and where local help is available. Call me old-fashioned, but I believe wholeheartedly in the power of what people can do when they come together and are empowered to help each other.

That's our focus going forward. How do we come together and empower individuals, families, and communities from the ground up?

We do it by building coherence.

We do it by changing the paradigm.

We do it with innovative disruptions.

And we do it together.

CHAPTER 5

The Warp and the Woof in Balance

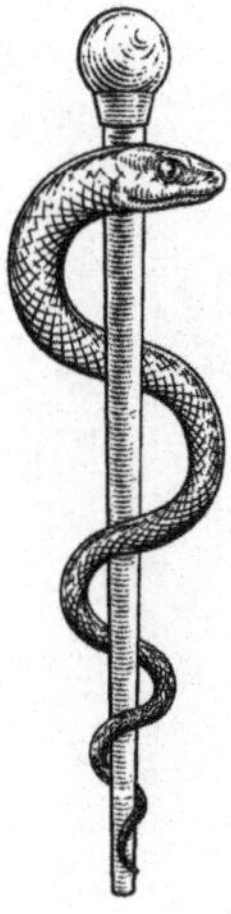

People like to blame a bad guy, and it sure looks like the bad guy in this case is the path of self-interest, the warp in the fabric of society. But both the warp and the woof are part of the big picture of health for individuals and societies. If it were not so, evolution would have closed off one of the paths by now. You can't blame people for taking the warp path of self-interest when it's one of the options available to them in an environment created by natural selection and random mutations that affect everyone equally. Nature is a neutral arbiter, maintaining balance between all competing interests—that's the model she's given us to follow, and there is an evolutionary advantage for self-interest in small groups.

The problem occurs when you get to larger and more diverse groups where the self-interested leaders of the small groups cannot command the fealty of the larger group. The imbalance created by the "natural selection" of self-interest by elements in the group that profit locally does not work outside the high walls of their basin of interest. If humanity is to truly follow the science and use evolution to guide the development of civilization, restoring balance to the larger society must be our highest priority, and it begins with busting the myths perpetuated by Social Darwinism.

Social Darwinism is when the fitness landscape is switched from the survival aspect of evolution to that of hierarchical power over others. It is the result of conscious evolution in the wrong direction.

Neoliberalism is its economic offspring. It creates walls around how we think by making us accept the lie that we are served best by allowing unfettered self-interest to rule the marketplace. For a civilization like ours, the marketplace is where ideas, products, and memes meet reproduction—reproduction being the final step that assures proper evolution. And if the process is imbued with the moral base that Adam Smith based his marketplace on, his invisible hand will be just as powerful and successful as evolution.

In a system as complex as a large civilization, it's the only way we can follow nature's example and create the necessary balance to sustain us. We allow the wisdom of the collective to emerge based on choices that make individuals more fit in the marketplace, and doing so makes us *all* more fit. That's how we balance the warp and the woof.

But our current ruling paradigm favors the warp over the woof. It hogs novel ideas and innovations and slaps a price tag on accessing them, like when a drug company patents a medicine and you end up paying $1,000 per month for a drug such as insulin that costs $10 to produce. That's unnatural.

It's unnatural to manipulate people by making them choose from among options that only favor the ruling paradigm, like when election day comes and we are faced with the same two choices, democrat or republican, and most of the time it's not going to make a real difference in the end which one we pick.

Across the board, most of the choices available in the marketplace are *unnaturally* selected, and to a large degree we can blame our culture for this state of affairs. The warp elements of market opacity and money behind advertising are the large determinants of our fitness landscape. The institutions profiting from the current paradigm and *warping* the culture to serve their desires are the defenders of that status quo. As long as they control how we think and the choices available to us, the warp will continue dominating the woof.

On the other hand, the new paradigms of defense medicine and salutogenesis elevate individuals and community to greater importance the money because the science clearly shows that *true evolutionary fitness is found within healthy groups*. Changing our paradigm is how we change the culture, so start with yourself and talk it over with those close to you. Expose the lies of self-interest for what they are, while respecting that the people you speak with can and will make their own choices. Knowledge truly is power, and the knowledge you are gaining in this book and sharing with your community carries the power to affect change. Changes that bring true benefits will spread naturally, we just need to expose the lies by getting the right information out there, beginning with a better understanding of how evolution really works.

It's a huge challenge. This information is blockaded by the abuse of power, the walls around our minds, the manipulation of public discourse, and the lack of community, understanding, and control.

The old paradigm's warfare thinking, influenced by Louis Pasteur's misunderstanding of our relationship with microbes, is unhealthy. Making America healthy again means following the example of Claude Bernard, who exposed the error in warfare thinking and gave us instead the understanding that health begins with defense. For our purpose, defense is more than just physiological. It includes the elements of coherence—control, understanding, and meaning—that help us all be healthier in body, mind, and spirit. They include protecting the mind and arming the population with information. Each of us individually must make our choices, and if enough of us make good ones, the marketplace will spread the benefits to everyone participating in society. It's how to conduct a counter-insurgency against the forces that hijacked evolution, not by fighting, but by addressing the underlying issues and restoring one of the greatest discoveries in the history of science to its rightful place.

It all comes back to the relationship between the individual and the community. The community is the soil we all grow in, so now we will explore this relationship.

THE INDIVIDUAL

Written above the entrance to the temple of Apollo at Delphi is the maxim: "know thyself." It seems simple enough, but those two words carry a deeper meaning known to the Greeks who thought deeply about life, explored its mysteries, and came to understand "thyself" as more than just the ego. We are a part of something larger: a family, a community, a culture, a state, the human family—and are even children of, or a part of, God. Who we are is something greater than our ego, and that greater part of us needs to be making our choices.

Who we are is really not that different from particle physics. Photons, or light, are either a wave or a particle, and apparently there's a choice in the matter because the end result depends entirely on the questions we ask. So, too, we have a choice in who we are. Jerry related a story to me that exemplifies this. At one point in her life she was near death and had one of those experience where she left her body and wandered the halls of the hospital. Her mother had just left from visiting her and was going home when she abruptly made a U-turn and rapidly returned to Jerry, demanding that "you get back here." Jerry was obedient to the call and asked her mother how she knew she'd left her body. Her mother replied, "I've been there and know the territory."

Waves can probably do that.

Instead, we think of "thyself" as the ego, but the ego is a construct of perceptions, a fact known and taught by all major religions and schools of psychology. It's transient, meaningless, and not real—but the Thomas Rule about self-fulfilling prophecy makes it real. We mistakenly equate the ego with the individual and, believing it to be true, end up making it so.

Earlier, we talked about the two-choice survey created by Todd Rose to expose the collective illusion that everyone else will choose ego-driven self-interest over the greater interest of a self-fulfilling life; and we discussed the distinct probability that many respondents likely saw their pursuit of financial success as self-fulfilling. The ego is the reason why we don't see beyond that wall around our thinking. Therefore, we end up pursuing wealth and success instead of personal fulfillment, and in the end discover that it's all for nothing. "Vanity of vanities" is how the richest man of his time, King Solomon, pegged it.

Simple logic tells us that our individual choices and actions should balance with our collective interests. All actions come from individuals. All novel ideas—the mutations of society—come from individuals. The question is why a particular person chooses a particular action. And the answer, again, comes down to the warp and the woof. The warp path of ego domination produces self-centered people. It produces the competitive orientation that psychologist Michelle Dresbold's handwriting analysis found to be prevalent in particular among men like Donald Trump. It stands in stark contrast to the orientation centered on community found to be prevalent among networking women.

The greater self is too complex for the ego, and the ego is too limited to navigate through the illusions. That's the lesson found in the story of Narcissus. When his mother was pregnant with him, she asked the seer Tiresias about her unborn child. He told her that her son would thrive as long as he did *not* know himself.

Narcissists, like Trump, see themselves exclusively as ego; there is no consideration of their larger self, and they thrive by their self-interest. To know thyself means to know your *greater self.* In the story, Narcissus ends up seeing his reflection in a quiet pool of water and falling in love with it, blinding him to all else. He falls in love with his own image.

Throughout history, people have lost their way by fixating on the illusion of themselves as only an ego. Religions teach the difference between the ego and the greater self, but society doesn't.

The story of Narcissus is also a cautionary tale about collective illusions and how society transmits them by acting as the mirror that reflects the ego, not the greater self. For all of us, the slower, more deliberate and logical System 2 thinking processes predominate in safe environments, but outside of our safe places we are more reactive. We see ourselves reflected in comparison to others, and comparison is what the ego feeds on. For example, IQ scores would be meaningless if not for the comparison between scores. Score higher than average and the ego thinks itself a genius; score lower and it thinks itself deficient. That mirror lies, and if we look into it too deeply it transfixes us. We forget who we are and join the collective illusion.

The Haudenosaunee (Iroquois) "Thanksgiving Address" proposes that we live as part of nature—as participants in the democracy of the species—and we all share its bountiful resources.[64] Or, as in the Genesis story, we are given dominion over all, but to the Haudenosaunee, dominion means governing, or stewardship, rather than owning. The ego wants to own. The greater self known to the adepts at Delphi wants to steward.

Carol Lynn Pearson wrote a poem titled "The Steward" that takes the reader into the lives of an elderly couple about to retire from the farm and move into a condo in town. The husband looks at the farm and, satisfied, is happy with what a lifetime of work has built. The wife is at home cleaning the closets and okay until finding her violin in storage and recalling how she loved to play it and wanted to travel to town to play in the symphony. However, the farm came first and the violin second, and the husband did not notice:

"The shrinking of her borders. The drying up of her green."

He stewarded the land, but a truly good steward *actively* cares for everything in his or her domain—and people come first.

An important part of stewardship and governing means recognizing the value of counterwill in the citizenry and reducing it by giving them a meaningful say in their own lives. Otherwise, like the wife in the poem, they recede and dry up. Governing also means power, and power is catnip for the ego. The antidote for this weakness is stewardship instead of ownership, greater self instead of ego self.

Within communities, individuals live, work, and play, and if we follow the thinking of the Haudenosaunee and others, community interest is the lens through which we view all individual actions. But where is the line between community interest and infringement on individual liberty? To answer that question, we need to understand the nature of power.

In nature, power is based on maximizing control over both the environment and others. Females of all gendered species look for a partner who can protect them and their offspring, and they gain the best protection by mating with dominant males. This reproductive success ensures the continuation of the quest for power, but the quest tends more to the self-interest, virulent path than the cooperative, commensal path. The commensal pathway is when power is combined with love and in the service of justice, as explained earlier by wise men, from Confucius to Martin Luther King. We survive together, and to do that we must cooperate. This is the path of commensalism.

During our prehistory of hunting and gathering, leadership capacity and hunting ability determined which individuals dominated the group. Then, with the rise of agriculture, hereditary power based on a combination of economic strength and strength in numbers took over. Might makes right—the right to rule. It created inequality, but don't go crying to the person with the right to use might against you. Bad idea. To survive, you keep your complaints to yourself and learn the survival tactic of fawning—of swearing fealty until you can marshal your own forces of insurrection. Or it can also just lead to the learned helplessness that circles us back to where we are today, a society of individuals who have adopted learned helplessness as the best means of survival.

Learned helplessness is defined as "the belief that we can't change the course of negative events—that failure is inevitable and insurmountable."[65] It is a type of freeze response. I see it commonly in people who accept a doctor's diagnosis as if decreed by God, and it becomes a self-fulfilling prophecy. Learned helplessness is also a major factor behind why so many people choose not to vote. Why bother if it doesn't make a difference? Not voting is also a freeze response, and like other decisions made with the lizard brain, it leads to undesirable results in the long-term. The bad actors in and around the government get the message that there are no consequences for committing abuses. We end up with a government that becomes a threat and makes people prone to the false promises of autocrats.

"Drain the swamp" is a glaring example of desperate voters falling for the con. It caught on because people were seeing that years-worth of dark money injected into politics—billions upon billions of dollars—created conditions of corruption in the national government. Along came Donald Trump and his made-for-television strongman persona, presenting himself as the sort of outsider who could crack the whip on corruption. Enough people fell for it to elect him, the biggest desperation move in American electoral history, and once he grabbed real political power he immediately set about enriching himself and his wealthy backers, making the swamp deeper and raising the art of grifting to never-before-seen heights of abuse. And his backers, the avid religious right, provide the power at our primary elections to threaten hesitant politicians with their positions in government unless they also swear fealty and opt for learned helplessness.

Yes, he did get rid of some government programs, but you don't drain a swamp by cutting down its trees and swatting its flies. Money is the murky fluid of the swamp, and you drain it by removing the money from politics. It was a pipe dream to think that someone who had spent his life pursuing wealth was going to somehow be immune to its allure. No one in American politics has found a way to address this problem, though we think that the Wilderness Rules about how to wield power are a good start. People invested with power to make decisions for all of us need to be the most moral and ethical and I daresay wise, too, especially about the difference between the ego and the greater self.

Learned helplessness is about responses to failure, *not* to success. Learned helplessness is a control problem, *not* a competence problem. Martin Seligman is the psychologist whose animal experiments showed how it works in people.[66] And our CIA was quick to pick it up and use it in their e*nhanced* interrogations, despite bordering on torture. He atoned for the abuses of his research by helping soldiers with PTSD and their feelings of helplessness stemming from surviving combat after seeing their buddies killed and maimed. While that sort of trauma tops the scale in severity, there are lessons for all of us found in how Seligman taught his clients to "own the crap." Taking ownership puts a person into the position of being the rider on the elephant. Learned helplessness is a control problem, ownership establishes control, and Seligman provided daily exercises to make them aware of the power they had to affect their environment.

Those exercises start with noticing and writing down three things that happened during the day that were good *and* you had a part in creating, then thinking about and writing down how those things can be repeated.[67] It delivers control to the individual, strengthens the pathways to the brain's cortex, and weakens the pathways of the reptilian brain.

The bottom line for individual action is that it be driven by the cortical rather than the reptilian brain and be done in cooperation with others in a "nothing about us without us" sense. Ideas are the evolutionary mutations in society, and they always occur in individuals. Beneficial ideas spread because they are helpful. They help the individual and hopefully the community as well. They balance the warp and the woof.

The spread of beneficial ideas is the commensalism of the human world. Virulence is the flip side, and based on what we've learned from microbes, it means that the community needs to protect itself from the transmission of bad ideas—like when Trump was banned from Twitter, or when his advisors told him he could not do what he wanted. He was constrained, not by the deep state but by his own people.

There's no practical way of stopping the virulence of outrage on social media as it exists today, so we need an innovation that allows for the transmission of beneficial ideas, minus the manipulation of tech companies, data harvesters and public relations tricksters. The healthy pathway for the development of civilization balances the rights of individuals with the needs of the community. The next emergent technology that follows that pathway will come into popular use because it first succeeds in the marketplace. Individual choice is actually the foundation for community success. Nature showed us how to strike that balance, and now it's up to us to put it to use.

THE COMMUNITY

Thomas Jefferson spoke of a need to go through cycles of revolution to replenish the spirit of liberty. The problem with revolutions, though, is they often end with a tyrant in control, or a charismatic personality takes power and turns autocratic. Napoleon's France is a prime example of revolution gone awry, as well as Chavez's Venezuela and Orbán's Hungary. Most autocrats gain power after or during a period of chaos, like what Steve Bannon wants to produce.

During the Middle Ages, Ibn Khaldun wrote about revolutions, and one takeaway is that evolution, while slower than revolution, is preferable because it is more peaceful, natural, and likely to follow the healthy path. While we are proposing revolutionary ideas and innovations and for people to band together in the name of fixing the problems in their communities and society, we're not talking about angry mobs storming the Capitol. We want to promote evolution, not revolution, and that is done most easily and safely done by playing with the fitness landscape.

Communities evolve toward greater coherence under the right conditions, and it begins by promoting health in all senses of the word. The revolution I'm calling for is the one that creates coherence.

People living together in society have conflicts and give their government the right to settle them. Historically, societies become more peaceful when their citizens give their government the right to implement justice, based on an understanding of the relationship between a people and their government. The British Common Law that the Founding Fathers imported to America began this new understanding. Before then, the idea of the individual, and the collective rights espoused in the Constitution, were all but unheard of.

Out of this revolutionary new understanding grew the idea that putting principled people in charge of government is a necessary condition for democracy, which is what the Founders tried to do, but even principled people can misread intentions. One of the most famous examples is British Prime Minister Neville Chamberlain's acquiescence to Hitler that produced the headline "peace in our time," but in reality it sent the message to Hitler that Britain didn't have the stomach to stand up to him. In America, we have Richard Nixon and Donald Trump as ready examples of those who gain political power and then abuse that power to maintain it, forcing intervention to stop them. Some leaders are not big enough to meet the demands of their time. It's why the courts that follow common law interpret law based on precedent instead of statute. The power behind statutes is too easily abused, especially when the people in power are unprincipled.

Another mistake happened when the Founders reasoned that limiting the right to vote to male property holders like themselves was the answer to preventing ill-suited people from rising to power in the

American republic. We can look back now and see how that decision put us on the road to plutocracy. The error was eventually corrected when voting rights expanded to all men, freed slaves, women, and Native Americans. However, throughout that same 150-year period between the writing of the Constitution and the expansion of voting rights to all people, powerful groups heavily influenced by the wealthy entrenched themselves inside the government, and it was too late to stop them by the time the voice of the common people gained enough strength at the ballot to have an effect.

Since Aristotle's time, the wealthy in a democracy have feared that giving political power to the poor would result in the poor rebelling and taking their fortunes. Neoliberals today broadcast the same fear, but fact is, the progressive tax policies they oppose had been in place for decades as the country prospered and the rich are still rich. Warp-inclined people chafe at what they see as robbery through taxation, but woof-inclined people see wealth inequality destroying the trust needed for civil society to function.

During the heyday of American democracy, as the people really came into their power after World War II and the Civil Rights Acts of the '60s, we struck a balance that few people were happy with but most everyone accepted, and the balance was built atop an electoral process that allowed all voices to be heard. Voting meant something, and we all knew it. John Lewis, in his farewell to the nation before he died, said: "The vote is the most powerful nonviolent change agent you have in a democratic society. You must use it because it is not guaranteed. You can lose it."[68]

But political campaigns in our country have relied more on advertising with its psychological gamesmanship, paid tricksters, repeated lies, and mass hypnosis, that have muddied up the atmosphere so that few really understand the candidates.

Bad actors, both foreign and domestic, targeted the voting process to destroy the public's trust in it. The reliability of the process of voting is assured by its diversity; every state sets their own process under the eye of Congress. If there is any competition among the states, it's on the reliability of the process. But while the Supreme Court has seemed to realize that racial gerrymandering was out of bounds, they have followed their originalist views on its political side. Since the Constitution says nothing about political parties, they turn a blind eye on the Guarantee Clause, which guarantees that every state will have a republican (meaning representative) form of government.

From our point of view, proper representation is what needs to be guaranteed. Every state legislature draws a map of legislative districts based on population, but now they also know the political party of every voter in the state, and when that information enters the process of deciding district boundaries it's called gerrymandering. In North Carolina, a state where voters lean slightly Republican, redistricting has led to a legislature dominated by Republicans who win elections through gerrymandering. With no checks on their power other than a few pitiful shots from the federal courts, they acted like mad scientists by turning their extremism into law and policy. It's a pattern repeated across the country as sophisticated political operators and their computer programs find and exploit vulnerabilities at all levels of government, to gain power in collusion with bad actors in both the private and public spheres.

The arguments of oppositional populists favor powerful plutocrats who hype up threats against the people from the government, activating our lizard brains and pushing people in a free society to fight back, including by arming themselves with military-style weapons. Ronald Reagan said we should fear the government bureaucrat who shows up at our door with an offer to help, and this sort of populist message mutated to become what we hear today about the "lying mainstream media" and "government takeover of the Justice Department," but they are all variations of the same fear-mongering. Belief in those lies drives us to look for a savior who claims to have the power to fix our problems. Then, that savior takes power and turns out to be just another self-interested plutocrat, or worse.

Making voting easier and more widespread is one of the strategies we can agree with to counter this threat. Australia, for example, made voting mandatory for all citizens, like jury duty, but it may not work in the US because of counterwill and the streak among many of us toward defiance. We'd like to see an option for "none of the above" added to the ballot to allow the expression of counterwill. We also like ranked-choice voting, a subject we'll cover soon. We need innovations to counteract the learned helplessness that's keeping people away from the polls and creating a vacuum of power that the plutocrats, special interests, and bad actors in society are only happy to exploit.

Learned helplessness can be created inadvertently, like when we provide foreign aid to countries experiencing famine by giving them our surplus wheat, but not teaching them to solve their own problems. The better option is to give them food for the short-term and the resources and control to produce their own food in the long-term.

In medicine, we create learned helplessness by treating patients with chronic diseases without finding ways for them to participate in their healing. It robs them of a sense of control when they need it most. By helping people with chronic illnesses find better ways of coping, we increase their social capital by raising their level of coherence.

We all suffer from learned helplessness in dealing with our plutocrat-controlled government and the money it is mired in. Nature's way of dealing with this is to increase mutations to find a new and better way. Libertarians propose removing social safety nets and letting the cards fall where they may, forcing people to be more resourceful. In theory it sounds like a good idea to shift the burden away from the state, but we need only consider how that policy worked out during the Irish Potato Famine. The British ruling class debated whether giving food to the Irish would create a "culture of dependency." A hands-off approach was adopted, and consequently about 12.5% of the Irish population perished. It's one thing to believe in the survival of the fittest but quite another to watch a million people die and argue that it's for the greater good. The warp (or some would say warped) point of view completely ignores the woof of cooperation, Christian charity, and the role of government.

But there's truth to the fact that social programs don't promote adaptation. Dr. Ruby Payne, an educator who studies the culture of poverty, argues that learned helplessness is common in our poor.[69] They think that the future is a roll of the dice and there's nothing they can do to make it better. The poor and the sick need the sense of control that allows them to play with their environment and adapt in healthier ways.

Control is central to coherence, and children may be our best case study. Provide them with a safe place and control over a manageable challenge and they will play with it until reaching an understanding. In many ways, what we learned as children can be the foundation for solving adult problems by applying the "sandbox rules." Rule one is to make it safe. Whether children or adults, people must first be safe both physically and psychologically before they can play. It means control, not learned helplessness. Rule two is to provide age-appropriate, challenging toys. For a child it might be a Lego set, while for an adult it might be a community survey. This leads to understanding. Rule three of the sandbox brings meaning into the picture: allow friends to join in. Such play gives children a sense of coherence and, in the words of Max Perutz of the Cavendish Labs, makes all children gifted and highly motivated.

Empowering our poor and chronically ill with a sense of control that deals with both counterwill and learned helplessness, sets them on a more cognitive pathway that leads to better health. It's the same model we use for helping children thrive. Empowering our population with a sense of control sets us all on the woof path, which improves social capital and leads to a better and healthier civilization. It may lead to the rescue of our commons as well by sharing power with the people who have been left out.

In a democracy like ours, good government begins at the ballot box, and for reasons we've discussed, our system of elections is not functioning as it should. We think solutions are within our grasp, and they're so intuitively right, even young children would agree with the following proposed fixes. It may be our best hope for restoring the balance between individual and community by making representative government work again, which in turn will make America healthy again. It is our best hope for saving our republic.

INNOVATIVE VOTING SYSTEMS

Ranked-choice voting (RCV) holds great promise for fixing our election system. Instead of an up-or-down vote, voters list their favored candidates in order of preference, ranking their choices from one to three and beyond depending on the number of candidates of any political party in the race. With more than two candidates on the ballot and the option to rank those candidates from first to last, voters gain greater ability to make their voices heard.

If no one gets a majority of votes to win the election outright, the candidate with the least number of votes is excluded and their voters' second choices are distributed to the remaining candidates. If that vote tally produces a majority for one candidate, they win. If not, the next candidate with the least votes is excluded, their secondary votes distributed, and the process continues until someone gets a majority. It's a clever way of using added complexity to give voters a greater say in who represents them in government.

There are several benefits with RCV. One of the major ones is it reduces election costs. Elections are expensive to run, and runoff elections are common. Primary elections, where one candidate from each party is chosen to run in the general election, are polarized and almost always won by the candidates with the most money and/or the greatest appeal to a party's hardcore elements. RCV eliminates primaries and always delivers the majority candidate.

Another benefit is that it tames campaign rhetoric. Sarah Palin lost a congressional race in Alaska in 2022 because her rhetoric was so hostile to her opponents that she did not gain many second places. Palin gained enough votes to win in a two-way race, but she was not the alternative choice of enough voters to give her a majority of voters after eliminating the last-place candidate. Predictably, Palin cried foul, but moderate voices in her party like former party chairman Michael Steele supported the process and the results.

Many voters reject the radical nature of partisanship that rewards extremism. RCV pushes candidates to make their campaigning more civil so as not to turn away voters who might pick them as their alternative choice. RCV does not favor the interests of the radicals on either side of the political fence, and it is now used in Alaska and a handful of other places because of voter initiatives.

That's what I call innovative disruption! We need innovation, but voter initiatives are frequently driven by fear and anger, and in some cases such tactical measures are not in our strategic interest. California's Proposition 13 was one such measure. It gave voters a way of voicing displeasure about rampant property taxes, but an increase in the wealth gap, underfunded schools, and a housing crisis were among the unintended consequences. RCV is one of the initiatives we can get behind, but the history of initiatives gone awry is a lesson in the need for caution.

Another benefit is that it allows for a greater variety of candidates. Our two-party system always fears the disruption of a third-party candidate when the polls are close. With RCV, that fear is unfounded, but with more alternatives it may turn out that one of them has enough second place votes to actually win. That is a distinct possibility, and it would very likely change the nature of our government to one of coalition, or that one or the other of the leading parties would need to consider accepting, as has always been done in the past, the policies of the alternative. RCV, by empowering alternatives, would tame the excesses of our partisan politics.

To summarize, RCV:

- Saves money. It requires one election per cycle, with no primaries or runoffs.

- Discourages overly negative campaigning because it makes candidates think twice about spitting on each other to win. Campaigns become more policy-oriented and less vindictive.

- Encourages more people from a wider swath of the public to run for office.

- Expands voter choice. Political parties control elections now, creating a narrow funnel of candidates that end up on the ballot. But under RCV, more people can run under a variety of policies and parties, and some of them are likely to win. On a national scale, if enough fresh, reasonable voices win, it could eliminate the power of the filibuster protecting special interests and lessen the polarization in government. Injecting more political parties into the mix dilutes the power of partisanship. Parties are weakened, but policy-making is strengthened and improved.

- Changes the winner-take-all dynamics that distort our traditional election system. In many elections where multiple candidates vie against each other for one seat, the winner gains less than majority support. RCV eliminates that by continuing through the tiers until one candidate has a majority, giving that person a mandate when they take office.

RCV addresses how to vote and how votes are counted. Currently, state governments control our voting system, and it is a hodge-podge of counties and precincts. In its favor, I would say that the variety in local voting systems is a major hedge against computer hacking of our elections, but experts point out that our voting machines are vulnerable. We need a better option, and I may know what it is.

A secure electronic voting system begins with a "smart" text-only device connected only to an off-line (not connected to the internet) server at the county clerk's office. The smart device is encrypted with a voter's fingerprint or face recognition for security, and security is established before, during, and after the person votes. The device is the person's connection to the government, and the government to the person. It can be used by local representatives to query their constituents, and vice-versa. This is an appealing asset for government at all levels, and if done with federal assistance it could be used to iron out some of the problems with our current elections, such as gerrymandering and voter suppression.

The server's program must be open-source and publicly available, and changes must be consensually approved by a committee of programmers. The technology would not only provide a means for obtaining information about political candidates and representatives, it would also give citizens a means of questioning them. This method of voting is simple and removes hindrances like traveling to a voting location. Most importantly, it enhances voter control and encourages participation. The initial expense of providing a device for every voter is less than the cost of a few cycles of traditional voting. Plus, it builds understanding and connects people to their government—and that is meaningful. To keep costs down, devices could be refurbished and recycled from older phones and tablets that otherwise end up in the garbage.

Implementing RCV with built-in, secure electronic voting and communication between the government and the governed would build coherence in all three of its areas, and that is how we build a more perfect union.

ENSURING THE ACCURACY OF THE VOTE

Voting in the US is a hodgepodge of state-regulated procedures where access is often limited by political or plutocratic biases. It needs to be uniformly regulated to ensure its accuracy and broadened to encourage civic participation. Opening the code to public scrutiny is the only way to stop the conspiracy minded and the secured location at the county clerk's office and with no connection to the internet assures its independence and reliability. Confirmation after voting by returning the marked ballot to the voter for confirmation and using an old, hack-proof technology like a tape drive for recording the vote would make it safe. If dedicated voting devices are not used, a paper trail is the only secure record, and I think it's our only choice until we can guarantee that electronic voting systems aren't hacked. No one has disputed Oregon's vote tallies, where vote-by-mail is universal and ballots are read by optical scanners.

In the absence of electronic voting, maintaining the accuracy of the vote means, first, securing our voting machines, attaching a tape drive to every machine and recording voter choices after they approve the accuracy. That would be as secure as a paper ballot, faster to count the vote, and a lot less expensive to implement.

Another way of securing the vote is by using fingerprint ID.

A fingerprint is more secure than the practice of signature verification and photo ID. In India, the use of fingerprint technology with smart cards for cash transfers to the poor reduced corruption by close to half.[70] We know it can be done, and if we are to secure the accuracy of the vote, these innovative disruptions are Heaven-sent—they deserve due consideration. The public would jump at this opportunity, I think.

States would likely balk at the change because it would undercut their power. But the public benefit would eventually win, and with that public pressure we would also see the expansion of initiative benefits like fair voting districts and easier registration.

These days gerrymandering, the creation of unfair voting districts, is a complex science fueled by voter information available in massive databases. The Constitution says nothing about political parties so an 'originalist' interpretation of the Constitution allows for political manipulation so that the redistricting party can maintain unfair political power. Such an originalist interpretation completely ignores the Federalist Papers, written mostly by the Constitutional fathers Hamilton and Madison, where partisanship and its problems are a major theme. A republic exists by the consent of the governed, and that consent should not be watered down through the gerrymandering that creates "safe" districts where one political party or the other is all but guaranteed to win elections.

A better solution for drawing voting districts is provided by topology, the branch of mathematics dealing with shapes and surfaces. 'Random walks' is a common tool mathematicians use to divide surfaces into segments, and it can easily be applied to population maps. If the random walk tool is population-based rather than party-based, it will produce the fairest and most coherent voting districts.

Gerrymandering is cheating to win. The political strategy behind it is clear, so it is not likely to be fixed from the top. That is why we need the courts to do their job. So far, they have bowed out, leaving it up to the people and their initiatives. Initiatives appear to be helping for the most part, but much more is needed, and twenty-four of our states do not allow voter initiatives.

THE COMMUNITY AND TRANSPARENCY

Transparency is not just good in politics, it's good in the marketplace as well. A *transparent marketplace* is the best way to manage any complex system because it empowers decision-makers. Today, the marketplace is anything but transparent. Joe Stiglitz argued that the "invisible hand"—Adam Smith's moral based guide that would ensure continued prosperity—died due to market opacity.[71]

In a complex market system, the consumer is the voter and is similarly empowered by information, but who provides the information? It's an important question for ensuring transparency because, as Adam said, when self-interested businessmen get together, they collude to profit off the people. Currently, the answer is mostly the self-interested businessmen, and if they are really self-interested, they will prefer that their customers remain blindfolded. Their advertising dollars provide most of the information. They pander to our survival-oriented behavior through outrage that demands our attention, or to our vanity and need to belong.

If the public demands more transparency and the business world does change to include the customer in their domain of interest, then the buyer is aware of a product's problems as well as benefits, both sides benefit. If the Boeing engineers who questioned the "Max's" flight computers were allowed a voice at the table that included the purchasers, lives would be saved, and more fit planes sold.

But sometimes transparency is harmful—like when it's coupled with outrage. A local story from my area exemplifies this dilemma. A group of first-grade students were able to escape classroom monitoring to engage in some sexual exploration. Several youngsters participated, and one of the participants recorded it, which led to its discovery. Child Protective Services investigated. Parents were notified and interviewed. The video clearly showed that no coercion happened and that no one was hurt; it was the kind of exploration and experimentation that children do in the Samoan "children's house," where innocence is presumed. But the aunt of a girl in the middle of the storm had a different view. She thought her niece was abused and injured, and she shared her outrage on social media. Fox News picked up the story, and reason flew out the window. I was made aware of the happening from a son who heard about it on Fox. A mob mentality took over. If the girl in question sustains any lasting damage from this incident, it will most likely come from the aunt's outrage, not the original incident. As the Samoans know, things that happen in the children's house are innocent and not talked about.

Using stories like this, tricksters, or just unaware helpful people manufacture mass movements, as happened with satanism and alleged abuses in day care facilities some years ago. Helpful therapists did not realize how well children read them and readily built the stories that the therapists were looking for with their questions. People join the flock and behave how the tricksters want. Information is weaponized in such an atmosphere of fear and threat, so we need to do more than just pick off a few of the bad actors. Only the mass education of the public to recognize the tactics used against them has any hope of changing the situation. The transparency needed here is through a better understanding of children and their development.

Interestingly, the tactics of the tricksters follow the same rules that Craig Reynolds used to program computers to mimic the flocking behavior of birds. Flocking begins with a threat—that's primary. Once the flock is formed the rules are:

1. Keep your distance from your neighbor.
2. Aim for the center of the flock.
3. Follow the flock in direction and speed.

In human behavior, these rules define a mob better than they do a crowd, and in this day of powerful computer software creating "deep fake" videos that can't be distinguished from real ones, it's easier than ever to use trickery to show a threat that forms the flock. While crowds have been touted as being wiser than individuals there are distinctions that make that so.

Edward Chancellor offers ideas on how to cope with this problem in his review of William Bernstein's *The Delusion of Crowds.*[72]

> Bernstein, drawing on James Surowiecki's *The Wisdom of Crowds* (2004), describes what's needed for a crowd to give accurate predictions or estimates: it should display "*independent individual analysis, diversity of individual experience and expertise, and an effective method for individuals to aggregate their opinions.*" (emphasis added)

In other words, the crowd should not be a mob driven by impulse, but a group of cooperating individuals. Chancellor continues, showing how a crowd moves to a mob:

> Errors appear when individuals become overly influenced by what others think. "The more a group interacts," Bernstein writes, "the more it behaves like a real crowd, and the less accurate its assessments become…. As put most succinctly by Friedrich Nietzsche, "Madness is rare in the individual—but with groups, parties, peoples, and ages it is the rule." [Charles] Mackay also recognized this; perhaps the most famous line in [his] *Extraordinary Popular Delusions,* is "Men, it is said, think in herds; it will be seen that they go mad in herds, while they only recover their senses more slowly, and one by one."

The madness of the herd is a form of mass hypnosis. Entranced, the herd can be directed and bent to the will of the hypnotist. You may enter a trace state and not recognize how vulnerable you are to suggestion. January 6th exemplifies this. Psychotherapist Ivan Tyrrell says of trance:

> Anyone who can focus their attention, who has a good imagination or who can become emotionally aroused, will, at many points in time, enter trance. We are in a self-induced trance whenever we are highly emotionally aroused in what is usually thought of as a negative way: anger, fury, hatred, fear, anxiety, worrying, depression, envy, greed, selfishness—all such emotions cut us off from our thinking brains and give us a locked-in, limited view

> of reality. The same is true when we are in thrall to conditioned belief systems that we cannot see beyond, whether those of religions, cults or politics. Exciting events which we experience as positive are no less limiting in terms of our seeing the bigger picture—however thrilling it may be to support one's team to victory, to feel swept away by music, to be moved by poetry, art or drama, to fall in love or make passionate love or experience an awesome wonder that takes our breath away.[73]

Trance states are a form of altered mentality; they open the brain to others and their suggestions and instill a desire to make those suggestions real. Trance and hypnosis happen subconsciously and, like Haidt's elephant, are hard to stop once they get rolling. And it is a mistake to think that hypnosis is only used in therapy. Scott Adams, the Dilbert cartoonist and a trained hypnotist, told host Bill Mayer in April, 2016 that Trump was going to win because of his proficiency at mass hypnosis.

Once you know how hypnosis works, you will see it being used against you all the time. The tools of mass media are powerful agents for affecting the mind. Hitler used mass rallies and loudspeakers. Roosevelt used radio broadcasts. Trump's following has been described as a social club where it's just plain fun to belong. It's all trance. By being aware of it and its power we can shift the paradigm to the healthier path for society, the woof, the rider on the elephant, which comes from the cognitive, strategic brain, where cooperation, and cooperative communication with others breeds coherence.

The people using trance and hypnosis to manipulate the masses know what they are doing is wrong, but they do it anyway because nothing is stopping them, and it gives them power and profits.

A common enemy provides both the threat and the direction. "We" are right, and "they" are wrong, like how Fox News did it with the "scandal" that took place in a first-grade classroom. This creates the perception that everyone believes a certain way, and if you want to be part of the flock, you must go that direction too. If you are on the left, of course you are going to support democrats. To do otherwise would mean you are one of *them*. If you are on the right, republicans are your people. Liberal versus conservative is a popular dividing line, and it all comes back to the ages-old human habit of treating everyone outside their flock as *the other*.

The media is increasingly aligned with the partisan nature of our politics. Social media does that on steroids. Both create basins of interest, paradigms that blind us to the reality of complexity that is the real world. They are just as much creators of opacity as the self-interested businessman.

They say that birds of a feather flock together, but it's mostly untrue. Most bird species will readily allow other bird species to join their flock. Strength in numbers is thought to be why they do it.[74]

COMMUNITY IMPLEMENTATION

The remedy for mass manipulation begins with understanding how our brains work, and with recognizing messages designed to trigger lizard-brain thinking. When exposed to triggers, take a time-out. A breathing exercise helps: count the seconds it takes to inhale and double that as you exhale. Doing that for just a few minutes calms your mind. See past surface appearance. Ask who benefits, who is pulling the strings, and who it hurts. All too often, our dehumanization of others is masked by virtue, as when Nixon started the drug war to target his political enemies. When we can have group discussions in safe places based on the arguing to learn format, which include a diverse population of those affected, the problems associated with reactive thinking disappear.

And it turns out that minds are changed, not by arguing, but simply by listening to others' stories—even others that are *other.*

Group discussion provides the *understanding* and the *meaning* necessary for coherence, but *control* is what guides them. Control is most often the missing ingredient to coherence, and coherence is the rider atop the elephant with a clear view of the surroundings. Education, good information, and experience provide the understanding that acts as an inoculant against manipulation and deception. More trust can be built for our government if the information coming to us is fair and just. But with profit-oriented plutocrats in control of our information sources, including government sources, our understanding can easily be warped.

At this point, our best hope is for innovative disruptions to emerge that are clearly superior for providing information to the public. It could be through technology such as social media, but we are encouraged by talk going around, past and present, about expanding public education to junior colleges and trade schools and instituting a national service program for all students after high school.

My term for this is Defense ed.; it is applying the same principles that are successful in medicine to our society, and its aim is to build the good soil (Bernard's term for our physiologic defenses) that our nation needs to survive. Civics would be central and college credit applicable. John Roberts recommended such courses in his 2019 year-end report. He wrote of how John Jay, our nation's first chief justice, was unable to continue contributing to the Federalist Papers because of an injury incurred while helping to quell a mob in New York.[75] Roberts pointed out that angry mobs egged on by rumors have no place in our society and today's leaders often argue the same. But the riot in New York was in response to graves actually being robbed to provide cadavers for anatomy lessons in the local hospitals, and authorities were doing nothing to stop it. Then as now, the best way to prevent mob violence is for the populace to maintain interest in, and understanding of, both the processes of government and the needs of the community. And if those needs are met by a black market, find a way to legitimize it. Mobs, whether in 1788 or January 2021, think as one—from their lizard brains—but groups of people looking for answers, as Roberts describes, think as individuals—from their cortices. That individual thinking is the difference between productive group thinking and a mob.

Making civics courses a focus in these moves and following the rules for building coherence, we could produce a generation of young adults inoculated against manipulation.

We see advantages to running such public service programs that provide free education after high school under control of our Department of Defense. It might help the DoD to expand its idea of what defense really is; fixing the cracks in society makes the nation stronger and more resistant to outside manipulation. It's Bernard's approach to making the soil healthier. The military is also the best example we have of successful integration along racial, ethnic, and gender lines. It took a while but they have done an admirable job eliminating the caste system, one of our larger cracks, from the military, so they might as well take on the task of doing that in our society.

And the accompanying military training would introduce another benefit—a likely decrease in mass shootings. We agree with the NRA's observation that few of the shootings are committed by people who have had formal training in the use of firearms, implying that such training might be effective for addressing this tragic problem. It would also give us the opportunity to spot people coming out of high school who definitely should not be armed, as well as some ability to address the reasons why.

The recommendation for such a program is congruent with Gordon Allport's *contact hypothesis.*[76] Allport, a prominent American psychologist and author of *The Nature of Prejudice,* argued—and numerous random trials have confirmed—that contact with people outside of your home group reduces prejudice if done correctly. Allport would make service to the country and attendance in civics classes mandatory. Classes would mix genders and ethnicities and use proven methods to build group cohesion: exercise, dancing, dining, yoga, Tai Chi, synchronized breathing—something everyone does together. These methods build group cohesion and a sense of safety, which is critically important for group success. The groups are challenged with controversial and divisive topics such as abortion, the role of human actions on climate change, conspiracies, and institutionalized racism. The goal is to strive for consensual decisions, ensuring that everyone is heard.

Roberts, Allport and others see civics education as a way to mend the cracks in our society—cracks created by systemic distrust of those seen as racial and ethnic *others,* or of those in power who are often targeted—correctly or not—for abusing that power, and whether in the marketplace or the government makes no difference. The absence of trust in civil society introduces toxic polarization and political mobocracy. Focusing on educating younger generations is more likely to yield results because they are not as far along the confirmation-bias pathway as the older generations, but many of us distrust our government, especially with the education of our children. To alleviate that fear, the civics classes must be transparent, with written explanations, and close and frequent ties to local newspapers making them available to the public. And the results of their consensual conclusions for the best path forward also need to be published locally.

Getting along with others is often difficult when we live in echo chambers filled with the kind of ethnically-targeted information Kevin Phillips found useful for manipulating elections, but a period of service to the country opens opportunities for mixed group discussions that can provide ways to overcome tribal isolation. Political scientist Chiara Cordelli writes:[77]

> Trust-generating relationships with people different from us provide distinctive arenas for the direct, informal, and safe experience of other points of view. This experience is generally necessary to fully exercise the capacity to confront and revise one's conception of the good. For example, adolescents who grow up in "segregated friendships" and lack meaningful bonds with a diverse set of peers often lack the capacity to engage in dialogue and deliberation with people different from them, as well as to revise the role models their parents impose on them.[78]

Derek Black is a case in point. Early in life, he followed in the footsteps of this father, a KKK Grand Wizard. Home-schooled Derek indoctrinated people his age through an online organization for kids based at Stormfront.org, his father's online hate group. His awakening came gradually after leaving home to attend a university in Florida, where his circle of friends included Jews.[79] He went on to advocate against racial hatred and bigotry, and his example confirms Cordelli's argument that exposure to others and their stories possesses real power to change one's values.

Derek's case also exemplifies the best approach to rescuing such people from their 'basin of interest' foxholes. Prior to his enlightenment Derek targeted his followers on a local Black minister. But the minister neither reacted in anger nor condemned him for his bigotry, and the two men eventually became friends and spoke publicly together about their experience. Such tolerance comes most forcefully from seeing who we are underneath our fragile egos. People whose egos are focused on arguing to win would condemn Derek, creating counterwill that would only succeed in keeping him entrenched in his prejudice.

Much the same as Derek happened to George Wallace after he was shot and paralyzed from the waist down. Shirley Chisholm, a black Congresswoman, visited Wallace in the hospital telling him, "I would not want what happened to you to happen to anyone." With that, the previously committed racist cried; tears that represented his move to a better paradigm. When he later, unannounced, interrupted a Sunday service to convey that message, his words were simple and contrite:[80]

> "I have learned what suffering means. In a way that was impossible [before the shooting], I think I can understand something of the pain black people have come to endure. I know I contributed to that pain, and I can only ask your forgiveness."

The congregation responded by singing Amazing Grace. Sometimes it takes a major trauma to wake us to the fact that we are all part of a larger community. And with that realization comes the understanding that the community we belong to should be the subject of our play with the fitness landscape.

I recently had a conversation with a local history professor who told me about his disciplines efforts to incorporate arguing to learn in the classroom. They found most of the students hesitant to argue, which they blamed on our political partisanship and the rampant use of social media to label people as *others.* I was thrilled by that type of interest since the need would be great should our nation adopt the civics courses discussed earlier, but I added the need first to build a cohesive group by some sort of shared play. While we are *homo sapiens,* we are also *homo ludens (playful),* and our play is often what brings us together. Arguing to learn is an exploration of that play that's mostly about listening. As many have pointed out, values are more important than facts in our mental makeup, and values *and culture* change as we listen to the life stories of others. Consensus is the aim. Consensus provided the governance of the Occupy Wall Street protests, and is the best way to ensure that all voices are heard. Consensus builds both understanding and meaning.

Consensus is also suggested to fix the Supreme Court's increasingly obvious political orientation. While many of its decisions are unanimous, those that aren't, tend to follow political orientation rather than sound legal reasoning. We think these decisions should be left up to the people, not partisan judges. We agree with David Orentlicher who wants a mandate for the Court to reach unanimous consensus on all decisions. [81] Cases where consensus is not reached would result in all sides writing a legal basis for their differing points of view to be sent to Congress as well as to civics classes around the country. And finally, if an accepted resolution is not reached, the issue would be put to the people.

Following the military example of "see one, do one, teach one," adept students at these civics classes should in turn be honored by local news and participate in community civics classes for the purpose of increasing our unity. Teaching the mixed benefits of both self-interest and cooperation would follow the pattern described by Jonathan Haidt (he of the elephant and rider metaphor) to resolve our tribal differences:

> If you put individuals together in the right way, such that some individuals can use their reasoning powers to disconfirm the claims of others, and all individuals feel some common bond or shared fate that allows them to interact civilly, you can create a group that ends up producing good reasoning as an emergent property of the social system.[82]

Haidt's requirements are easily established by giving the group a challenge to reach consensus on an issue. Such a format requires listening, understanding, negotiating, compromise, and giving a voice to everyone at the table. But Haidt overlooks the value of storytelling and the lived experience of others—these are more likely to change minds. Stories, more so than rational arguments, are the cooperative communication that led to *Homo sapiens'* evolutionary success, recognizing and reinforcing the idea that our values are more powerful than facts in our decision-making. The meaning part of coherence is built by listening to others' stories, which is why these small groups need a mixed structure.

Listening to the stories of people different from us opens us to changing our opinions. It's a lot easier, as Haidt implies, when the group is bonded in some way by participating, as discussed above, in activities together in synchrony.

Peter Coleman, a social psychologist at Columbia University interested in conflict resolution, argues that the disruption introduced by the coronavirus pandemic provided an opportunity to overcome our polarities. He points out that Costa Rica, after decades of civil war, intentionally disbanded its armed forces and shifted its focus to the environment, education, and health. That nation now ranks highly on peace indexes. Both Coleman and Clayton Christensen, the scholar behind the concept of innovative disruptions, agree that such discussions open the door to the resolution that leads to progress.[83]

Universal basic income is a proposal to send direct cash payments to those in need, to address income inequality, poverty, and economic security, but its flaw is that 'something for nothing' would engender large amounts of counterwill from taxpayers footing the bill. But tie the payments to a requirement for civic participation of some kind and we think it would be better tolerated. It would avoid the 'something for nothing' trap and be both wiser and fairer by rewarding the individual for their participation, which translates to some control and an *understanding* of civic responsibility, plus a *sense of meaning* from gathering with others in the community. Such meetings could be held at schools, churches, or places of employment—places where some group cohesion is already present. Diversity should be encouraged, and the meetings should be limited in size so that everyone has a voice as well as a seat at the table. The way to ensure a voice is to make decisions consensually; it's important for gender and ethnic equality.[84]

I know from experience that community is where we find answers. Years ago, a middle school counselor in my area expressed concern about the rising pregnancy rate at her school. She wanted to do something about it, but sex education classes were not state approved. I shared her interest and had access to a program that I thought would work. We presented it to the boys and girls, separately, in the 7th and 8th grades. Not only did the pregnancy rate plummet and remain there until the program crashed because of an indiscreet educator answering questions about homosexual practices too bluntly, but several cases of sexual abuse within the families of students were uncovered within days of the first group meetings. The success was because of the cooperation between the counselor and those involved. At another location, I saw the same need and approached the school district where sex ed classes were not banned, and they approved my program. But the middle school counselor saw it as a top-down infringement. Her counterwill destroyed the program.

Another personal example of community implementation comes from a nephew who works for the LAPD. While on light duty after an injury, he worked with a professional educator to provide alternatives other than joining gangs for the city's young men. He had grown up in a gang environment and knew what that community needed. Their program changed the course of many lives and demonstrated the power to affect change at the community level by empowering the people who truly understand its challenges.

My third example comes from my wife Jerry, who as a counselor and assistant principal collaborated with her elementary school principal, who recognized that children are already learning by playing with their toys long before they first step through the school doors, so why not continue that style of learning at school? Within two years, their innovations had lifted that school to the status of Mentor School, an example for all other schools in Texas. It was the first school in the state to be honored that way. Then, the principal was hired away, Jerry moved over to the high school, and two years later the school had lost its edge. Clearly, the empowerment at the school level, where people best understand its challenges, made the difference.

These three personal examples of individual actions in the community show the difference it can make. The alchemy that produces this magic begins with individuals who are not mired in self-interest, cross-pollinating with other individuals in the community, avoiding the generation of counterwill by initiating and running things locally, and more importantly bringing associates along with them by cooperative communication. And the point here is that nature provides the example of different species all working together, and while nature's cooperation took many years of evolutionary adaptation we can accomplish the same with cooperative communication and a wisely planned fitness landscape.

How, then, can we teach others to build their communities?

It begins with a problem, and the problem needs a forum in the community where it can be discussed to hash out solutions with people in the same room together. It could be provided by the community civics classes discussed above, and by churches. We wisely chose to separate church and state because of the lessons learned from centuries of religious wars in Europe, but our proposal piggybacks atop a role that churches have traditionally played, and it avoids the toxic mix of church and politics. The traditional role of religion is to look out for the poor, the widows, and the disabled. In our online world there are myriad ways to monitor a group's behavior so that religious groups that work to observe their traditional role are rewarded and encouraged. Cass Sunstein would call them nudges; they are both inexpensive and effective. It's what xylitol does to the affected microbes in our airways. It's a crucial factor that requires a bit of a history lesson to understand why it's so important.

Power had traditionally rested with the royalty and the church, but the advent of the printing press and public availability of the Bible threatened ecclesiastical power. Counterwill blossomed and wars followed. The Peace of Westphalia in 1648 ended ecclesiastical power and established sovereign political states, and less than a 150 years later, the US Founders followed that example for mediating the arguments between catholic Maryland, protestant Massachusetts, Quaker Pennsylvania, and so forth, which was a major source of distrust among the colonies. The Founders divorced government from religion but consequently ignored the murky fact that to organize along religious lines is hardwired in human beings. And that religion, with its focus on service to others, contributes greatly to the advancement of civilization, and is likely why religious states survive longer. To exclude religion from the picture because of its past and present quest for ecclesiastical power and the abuses that result is to throw out the baby with the bathwater. Today, we can support religions that in turn support their communities' civic programs aimed at welfare, the traditional focus of religious institutions.

Influential sociologists Alexandra Maryanski and Jonathan Turner say that "the very forces that pushed hominins to become more social, more group oriented, and eventually more capable of forming enduring ties among males and females to form the nuclear family *are the very same forces* that make religion inevitable in human societies."[85] If our churches shifted their focus back to their communities, these forces could again be applied to advance our societies.

I have seen the good it can do. The Mormon church in which I was raised has a welfare program that works, but its top-down orientation leaves no room for building a diverse community or passing control down to individuals. It is also friendlier to members than to outsiders. But the need for welfare is universal—most of us at some point in our lives could benefit from the help.

Resilience is another key factor in building communities, and the research shows that access to help builds resilience, and conversely, lack of access degrades it.

I learned this lesson personally after finding myself in need following a showdown at the local hospital where I worked. Its obstetrical department was poorly run, clearly resulting in an unnecessary fetal demise in one of my patients. That experience prompted me to write a letter to my obstetrical patients stating my intent to switch them to a neighboring hospital with a more reliable department. A few weeks later, an obstetrical disaster involving one of the other doctors raised the issue to the top of the list for the hospital and the doctors like me who trusted (or in my case, were losing trust) in it. At a staff meeting, without thinking of the legal liabilities it would load onto the hospital, I related my experience, my decision to switch, and the letter I sent. After realizing my mistake in being open, I understood the reaction of the hospital—I needed to be gone.

But my family did not want to go. We were living in a three-fourths completed home that was big enough for us, and we had friends in the community. There are many ways for a hospital to resolve an issue like this, including a buy-out. They chose instead to force me out. Over the next months a series of incident reports were collected on my presumed failures as a physician, and then I was told about them and put on probation. That's when my counterwill blossomed. I explained the errors in the reports to the medical board at a neighboring hospital, as well as to the state medical board, and convinced them of the politics behind the issue. But that did not affect the community; my practice dropped to non-working status, and I moved to doing emergency medicine elsewhere.

Bouncing back was not in the immediate game. I asked the church for help with food. They said, "go to your families for help first," an idea that angered me until I realized it was proper. My wife tried to help and encountered her own problems when she butted up against a recalcitrant culture in the LDS Church. She tried to put her PhD in Counseling Education to use in their social services and needed approval of the local Church authority. The individual representing the Church told her that she was better off staying at home to raise her family.

Friends came to the rescue with ways to sue, which eventually did work in our favor, but by that time we had left our home, moved elsewhere, and the hospital had closed.

The elements of my resilience were the same as those shared in this book. I had control in finding the errors in the reports against me and explaining them to outside authorities. I had others advising on tactics to gain recompense, other avenues of work, and family support. And when it finally came to a judge and jury, I had an exceptional nurse who had been around the block with hospitals that had chosen the same tactic—and talked about it. It's an example of pathological culture:

> In a pathological culture, crucial information about potentially damning errors or hazards is hoarded by those in power and often used as a weapon to silence critics.[86]

It's not exactly similar, but they silence whistleblowers the same way.

Help from others was key in my resilience.

The counterexample of the LDS Church in the above story is a very good illustration of the 'I know better than you' model of help. While family help should come before church or government help, we are not set up that way—it's not our model. So, the initial reaction, as it was in my case, is counterwill against someone above you telling you what you should be doing—and most of the time your counterwill is dismissed by the power and useless for you. Welfare critics say that such programs prevent people from progressing out of poverty, and they are correct. You don't have to look hard to find faults in any program managed in an environment full of complexity like a bureaucracy. Moving control down to the community is how you tame that beast, and despite the separation of church and state, local churches are the logical choice to spearhead welfare programs in their communities.

In the Black section of my town, the churches already fill this role. Made up of five small congregations, they monitor the needs of the community through a joint committee, and the first Sunday of every month the committee presents that information to the congregations. They then allocate resources donated by individuals able to help. They are not strangers from the government at your door offering help, they are friends offering a hand.

Welfare should come first from the family, but we would see a resurrection of church efficacy at the local level if our local ministers' groups combined forces to address community and family needs. And the need is not just for welfare but for safe places to come together and conduct the civics classes suggested by John Roberts. Such a move would require the integration of the churches similar to what we have done with our schools and military, making them less tribalistic. They would need government support to do that, but to move control of charity from the government to the churches would be a very healthy move.

The Good Samaritan, otherwise known as *caring for the other*, is an ancient religious practice that would go far in reducing the leeriness of church and state working together. Both church and state function to help the people, especially those in need. The wall of separation between church and state was very much needed when the Founders wrote it into the Constitution because churches were self-centered and tribal and corrupted by power—and many still are. But it is possible to use power wisely if church leaders understand and live by the Wilderness Rules, and perhaps a civics lesson or two would help them understand that separation of church and state is as much about protecting the church as it is the state.

Donald Trump exemplifies the downside of combining political power with the ecclesiastical power of the Christian right. To them, he is a messianic figure, but outside of that hardcore minority the perception is that some of the most religious people in the country played a large role in putting a malignant narcissist into the White House! That breach of trust can only be healed through a complete reversal, similar, but not necessarily as final, as that following good Friday two millennia ago.

GOVERNMENT CAN BE GOOD

Ronald Reagan was not altogether wrong to fear government largess. Politicians of his time worried endlessly about the abuse of state-funded help, but their political posturing about "welfare mommas" and whatnot did more harm than good. Government can be good when it offers help that builds the relationships that make a community, but it has no direct way of accomplishing that. Integrating public schools tried, but the effort got lost in the seven decades of counterwill that followed. Bringing down the walls that divide us is what our government tried to do, which ran into counterwill. A better way to deal with that problem would be to play with the fitness landscape as Singapore did as seen in Chapter Four. Building apartments with their proportional occupancy addressed the landscape and worked better.

Another idea from Singapore is their Central Provident Fund (PNF), a retirement fund like our Social Security, discussed more in our prequel. Lee Kuan Yew, the first prime minister of independent Singapore expanded and increased the funding for the program after the British started it. It can be used by individuals to pay for housing, education, and health care, and it can be shared among family members. Conceivably, it could be expanded to cover any other social good, such as food—with some kind of bonus for farmer's markets.

What a great program and model for Social Security to follow. We propose revamping Social Security and renaming it the People's Needs Fund (PNF), in homage to psychologist Abraham Maslow's hierarchy of needs. Maslow theorized that taking care of basic needs for shelter and food helps people create a safe place where the elephants are at peace and the riders can develop their higher capacities. Many argue that putting these funds under individual control would lead to abuses, and since it is also a part of one's retirement that's a concern worth considering. Coping with abnormal or potentially harmful abuses would be a good job for AI—and AI nudges in the right direction would be more helpful than any criticism. Studies by investment companies have shown that with the proper perks—financial incentives or variable interest rates—even the poor will fund an investment account.[87] With the information our government has on our financial situations, adding the needed perks would add a greater sense of control that would, in turn, facilitate people moving from Ruby Payne's poverty thinking with its learned helplessness, to the middle class thinking where one has a measure of control over their environment by what they choose to do. As pointed out earlier, this middle-class thinking is the foundation of democracy, and our middle class is being squeezed out of existence. It needs a boost, if not a lifesaver.

Sharing one's PNF within the family would make families stronger and social conservatives happy. And rather than a child benefit on the tax rolls, every child would get a grant from the government at birth to start their own PNF. Sharing within the local community (faith, school, city, or occupational, *not virtual*) would empower community-building and promote the idea that charity begins locally. Somewhat like what the Black community is already doing in my area of Texas; a small monthly transfer from an individual's PNF to that of their church would help satisfy community needs in a far friendlier and more effective manner than our current welfare programs.

Unlike other retirement funds, a PNF would give control to the individual instead of the bureaucrats who run Social Security.

It would also provide a direct means of government support where needed, bypassing the graft associated with block grants where only a small percentage gets to the needy.

Of the myriad ways we have to pay for healthcare, a Health Savings Account is the most practical. It's the only one that involves the patient (the consumer) in the marketplace where they can decide whether the treatment recommended is worth the expense, as well as being pressured toward healthier habits. As outlined earlier our current trajectory of healthcare costs is not sustainable. Defense medicine is the innovative disruption that can resolve that issue and return health care to the realm where, with insurance to pay for emergencies, it would be manageable with an HSA. A study from the libertarian-funded Wisconsin Policy Research Institute shows that empowering the patient in this way results in significant savings over third-party payment by health insurance companies, without a noticeable decrease in health.[88]

The formula is simple: give people more control to provide for their basic needs, rather than providing those needs for them and pushing them toward learned helplessness like we currently do in the US.

Unmet needs for the basics in life can drive people into a corner and make them desperate for solutions. We saw that process play out as Hitler brought Germany out of the Depression and the financial straight-jacket imposed by financial reparations stemming from World War I, and the same kind of process seems to be at play in the U. S. after manufacturing went overseas. The decline in our life expectancy contributed to by mid-life overdoses tells us the same thing. Do something different!

REFORMING THE EDUCATION SYSTEM

Our well-read and literate Founders provided the young nation with a strong impetus toward education because its benefits were obvious, but the government took no role in public education until many decades later. Parents, churches, and communities determined how children were educated. Education rose in importance in part as a response to the fact that historically, the clergy had a monopoly on education. As some of the only people who could read and write in a community, they maintained ecclesiastical power in the colonies. Knowing that, it's easy to see why the Founders separated religion from government, but the degree of separation went too far. Both government and religion function to build healthy communities and citizens, and nudging churches to do their part at the *local* level, where they can do real good, should not be prohibited.

As the young country grew, so did education. School funding came mostly from parents. New England led the way in making education a priority. Starting in 1837, Horace Mann used his power as secretary of education in Massachusetts to adopt a Prussian-style education system, which was considered the best of its time, and to this day we continue many of its traditions. After being elected to Congress in 1848, Mann helped to spread the Prussian system throughout the states. Based on universality, non-sectarianism, and curriculum, it became the basis for elementary school education, but its flaws soon became apparent.

The Prussian system is regimented, with children sitting still for long stretches and listening to their teachers. It's not natural. We forgot how children learn to learn. Newborn infants must learn how to work their bodies and get their needs met—at the same time—and they do this by trial and error, watching caregivers' responses and adapting—learning—in ways that gratify both infant and parent. Infants learn by playing with their environments, and it works well for them. Those pathways in their brains are myelinated and develop into what you might call learning freeways. By the time children enter preschool, their learning curve is almost vertical as they learn how to manage their bodies and interact with their environments. They are supercharged learning systems.

Then they run up against the Prussian education system. Expected to sit still and pay attention as the Prussian model dictates, the learning curve flattens. The children who can't hack it are labeled as having ADHD because they want to move around and play, the learning style that's myelinated in their brains. So, they are given suppressive drugs, supposedly to help them, but if their so-called hyperactivity is a symptom that indicates a problem, what does suppression accomplish? It's akin to bloodletting as a treatment for the inflammatory response. Some children adapt to the "sit still and be quiet" model of learning, but inwardly they rebel, and eventually their ability to control themselves collapses. It may end in a trip to the principal's office for disciplining, or in violence or suicide.

Today, the Prussian system is not the only game in town. Private education is an escape for those who can afford it, and home schooling for those that can't, or don't want government interference. In Montessori schools, play is still recognized as an important part of learning. The founder of Amazon, Jeff Bezos, enjoyed a Montessori education in preschool and thought so highly of it, he funded a grant program to open Montessori preschools in under-served areas. We are all wired for the exploratory style of learning, which raises the question of why we ignore what we know to be true and continue doing things to the contrary. Schools in general would work much better if all children could enjoy a play-based education, like the one Jerry helped to build in our community.

In education as well as any system dealing with living subjects, enhancing coherence and eliminating counterwill should be the guiding principles. Early in her career, while working on her master's degree in education, Jerry took a statistics class from a gifted teacher who used play in his class to try to break a slump in student scores on the statistics portion of the state accreditation exam. He divided the class into groups that rotated weekly so that all the students at some point would interact with each other during the term. At the beginning of each week, he gave each group a subject to learn about, and at the end of the week they explained it to the rest of the class. As a result, Jerry achieved a perfect score on the statistics portion of the accreditation exam, and her fellow students also excelled. Why? For the same reason that children—and all people—do better when given a sense of control and enabled to play with the learning material. Understanding follows, and working together as a group adds meaning to the experience. The mixing of students enables them to teach each other and use the knowledge and abilities of the group to help individuals overcome their deficiencies. Scientists in the right environments follow this learning pathway, too, though they may not know the science behind the reasons for it. We remember 5% of what we hear and 10% of what we read, but in group learning situations we remember around 50%, and if we use what we learn soon after learning it, as many students in Jerry's class did by teaching their classmates, retention soars to 75% to 90%.

We know how to improve the education system. We know how to improve government. We have the data, the studies, the policy papers, and the firsthand experience. The costs to implement these forward-thinking ideas are negligible. America was founded on innovation. The time has come to renew that spirit and bring all parties to the table to make it happen.

Chapter 6

Our Government

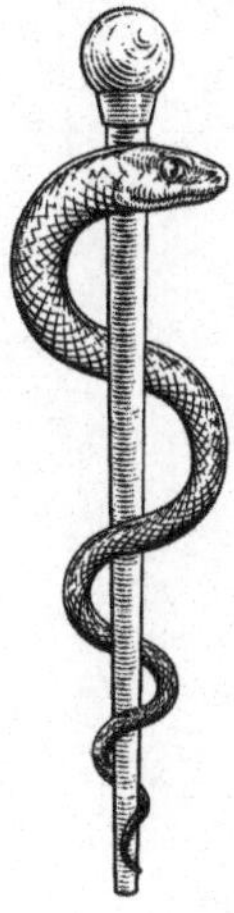

"The commitments that bind us to the social body are obligatory only because they are mutual; and their nature is such that in fulfilling them one cannot work for others without at the same time working for oneself."

–Jean-Jacques Rousseau

In one simple yet powerful sentence, Rousseau stitches together the warp with the woof by combining self-interest with group interest, because what is good for the group is good for the individual. The rising tide lifts all boats as long as our concern is as much for our neighbor's boat as it is for one's own.

The combination of self-interest with group interest produced amazing results for the nation. Alexis de Tocqueville, the French sociologist who toured America five decades after its founding, saw firsthand its rapid growth driven by individualism and community interest. He marveled at how quickly communities sprung up and built the elements of social capital: the schools, the churches, and even the bars and taverns that brought people together. Around the year 2000, Harvard political scientist Robert Putnam looked again at communities in America and saw them declining because its people are increasingly disconnected from friends, neighbors, and democratic structures.[89] His critique sparked a resurgence of interest in community-building. Communities build social capital, the fabric of social interconnection that we call the woof. Social capital is the value a society builds and stockpiles as people create a common bond by sharing stories and learning to care for each other. The cooperative communication that gave our ancestors the edge is also a large part of the coherence that leads to better health, both individual and social. To understand why America's social capital is depleted, we must first look at how it was built in the first place.

If you were there for the conversations the Founders had about the nation they wanted to create, you would have heard them talk about their greatest fear: creating a monarchy. So, a decade before writing the Constitution, they spelled out their vision for the new republic in the Articles of Confederation and deliberately avoided creating an executive branch of government. No executive branch meant no chance for an autocrat enthroning himself atop the government. Ten years later, after winning independence, they wrote the Constitution, creating an executive branch with the task of enforcing the laws, but only after creating a legislative branch with the power to keep the executive in check. In their minds, an executive was only needed to enforce the laws in oppositional states like Massachusetts, where the rejection of federal script—payment for Revolutionary War veterans—led to the Shays' Rebellion. Then, in Article III, the Founders created the judicial branch to act as an arbiter. Any civil duties not listed in the Constitution were left to the states. It's truly a visionary way of putting together a government by balancing political power, but its flaw is it does nothing about economic power. Its openness to abuse of the commons by the self-interested went unchecked until the progressive era, and by then the government had already been sold. Congress did nothing to stop the abuses, leaving it to the executive branch to reap the counterwill from the self-interested abusers. Counterwill that with the readily available adaptations rapidly grows into a bureaucratic society where growth and novelty are often put in a limbo of frustration.

Article IV defines the relationship between the states and the federal government. The states and their communities are where one can play with novelty and promote a generative system, using information for the benefit of all. The government is responsible for ensuring that states maintain a republican form of government, but it failed from the get-go by excluding slaves and natives from citizenship, then later, once that mistake was corrected, by allowing abuse through partisan gerrymandering and other methods of limiting the vote. As a result, we've ended up with what the Founders tried to avoid: an oligarchic form of government disguised as a democracy, run by the wealthy for the wealthy. So, what did they really have in mind when they created the government of the new nation?

CULTURE AND GOVERNMENT

As the Founders hashed out how to form a government, the biggest decision they faced boiled down to the power it would have. On one side of debate, Thomas Jefferson and his camp called for an agrarian economy of gentlemen farmers and decentralized government. On the other side stood Alexander Hamilton and his camp calling for industrialization and expansive powers centralized with the federal government. The debate is summed up as *states' rights vs. federal rights*, and it's not as much about determining who leads as it is about where they lead, how much power they need to get there, and what kind of society is best for the people.

Hamilton's side won and set the nation on a course of industrialization and centralized power in the hands of the federal government, seen at the time as a necessity for promoting trade and treaties with other nations. His vision resulted in creating the strongest economy and the wealthiest nation in world history, at the expense of following the warp pathway of self-interest over community interest. The defectors in the Prisoner's Dilemma game want unfettered capitalism, (i.e. opaque, as in those able to wear Gyges ring) in a mixed economy because it produces tremendous wealth and power concentrated in the hands of the few, despite how it leads to inequality and disaffection among the people. Sound familiar?

Predictably, the masses who got the short end of the stick periodically revolted. Following the Civil War, rapid industrialization led to monopolies, and a weakened nation succumbed to the opportunistic infection of robber baron capitalism. Monopolies such as Standard Oil, created by John D. Rockefeller, produced extravagant wealth and power at the expense of the majority, making the situation ripe for a big, fat counterwill response from the body politic to cleanse itself of its infection. Blood was spilled during revolts against the conditions created by industrialization and the monopoly of wealth and power. It got the attention of the wise leaders of the time, and leading up to World War I, Progressive politicians were voted into power with a mandate to break up monopolies and police the abuses. They promoted evolution over revolution and saved the government from being overthrown.

Along with the Progressive movement came the introduction of class warfare and communism, which were effectively countered with the creation of labor unions that gave workers some control in the workplace. However, closer to our day neoliberal policies squelched union power, so our position today is very similar to where we stood at the end of the 19th century, except we have little chance of electing people to office who stand up for the people, and the ones who do manage to get elected have little power to affect change with a Congress bought by the wealthy.

This issue is real, and the Founders were not altogether wrong in their appraisal of the masses and the need to protect the government against their worst impulses. As Christopher Achen and

Larry Bartels point out in *Democracy for Realists: Why Elections Do Not Produce Responsive Government*:

> Unfortunately, if there's one thing that history has taught us, it is certainly this: popular opinions are often little more than delusions.[90]

It's the point of view of people who see a nation that has excelled because of self-interest and Social Darwinism. The popular opinion of the folk theory of democracy—the belief that the people will elect candidates who reflect their wishes and desires—is one such delusion. Achen and Bartels conclude that neither politics nor democracy are rational, and solutions will not come from a new theory of democracy.[91] So what do we do now?

The democracy they describe is one stemming from campaigns that get our attention every four years when about 60% of eligible voters actually vote. In the off years non-presidential elections, it drops to 40%. We believe that the combination of expanding the House representation to what Washington wanted (1/35,000) and the establishment of civic discussion groups promoted by our legislators and conducted by our military would generate a much wider interest in our democratic system. Add to that the tablets that make voting easier and provide a personal means of interacting with our government, and we could empower our citizens to see a view other than super PACs and social media partisanship.

We are in desperate need of the generative type of society that sees its problems and weaknesses and that comes together to find ways to resolve them. What we have is a pathological system discussed earlier, where information is kept hidden and used in threatening ways to prevent progress.

The Tulsa Massacre of 1921, when a thriving Black community in that city was burned to the ground, was largely unknown for many years after it happened. Fear kept the victims silent. Guilt and power kept the perpetrators silent. And like the massacre in Tiananmen Square, the powers sat on it for as long as possible.

That story is similar today with critical race theory. We don't want our children to feel any guilt from their heritage but hiding it does not heal the wounds. Instead, what if we had a period of public confession modeled after South Africa's Truth and Reconciliation? That is a beginning, but it need not be public. We must come to realize that our lower castes have been treated wrongly and are in need of recompense. A personal *cognitive* recognition of being wrong is sufficient if it is followed by *changed behavior.* Even that can be challenging; it means radically changing one's life. The Apostle Paul did it on the road to Damascus, Derek Black did it in Florida, George Wallace did it in his hospital bed.

In our system of punitive justice, we see lots of sins that need to be punished, but God sees mistakes that can be corrected. Correcting them is done by the rider on the elephant, usually triggered by a story or a listener. It does not come from the ego centered lizard brain down below where the focus is on justifying the error. Cognitive therapists use a simple way of redirecting a person's thinking from their fear-based lizard brain to their cognitive brain by snapping a rubber band on the wrist. It "snaps" you back to cognitive thinking by sending a sharp signal through the nervous system.

In the long run, the solution is to recognize the differing values in self-interest and community interest. Evolutionary processes created them for our survival—both of them—but only one has become a problem.

Kondiaronk, discussed earlier as the native American behind the Noble Savage, saw this problem: "What kind of human, what species of creature, must Europeans be, that they have to be forced to do good, and only refrain from evil because of fear of punishment?"[92] He notes that his people don't have laws because they don't use money, and his ancestors lived contentedly without it, preferring a barter system.

But we remain a society where defectors ruled by self-interest have the edge, and those with financial power now control the political power, which is the definition of oligarchy. To those looking at our social classes it is this group see itself as entitled, not the people on public assistance. Power equates to survival under the rules of Social Darwinism and their view is that they deserve to rule. In human groups, it is usually the person who controls the most wealth or inherits their power through a dynasty. They defect because no one is stopping them, and they certainly aren't stopping themselves—they are entitled. It is leading to autocracy, which is exactly what the Founders feared and wanted to avoid.

It looks unstoppable, but solutions are within our grasp by restoring the balance between self-interest and group interest. A second populist movement is needed now to push power down to our communities and out of the hands of the gorillas.

MY FELLOW AMERICANS

To paraphrase a popular 1970s TV show, we can rebuild—we have the technology, the capability, the know-how. The show is *The Six Million Dollar Man*, a quaint sum these days—*only $6 million?* But perhaps the lesson here is that a little can go a long way when the funding is entrusted to communities and their leaders and organizers who know best how to invest and spend it. We do not need more government, better experts or stronger leaders, we need stronger and better communities.

It's how microbes have survived for billions of years on this planet. Alone, they quickly whither, but together, they have stood up against the most sophisticated weaponry medicine can devise. And if we keep hammering away at them, they may just respond in self-defense by mutating into something so virulent, there is no defense against it. The microbes are winning the war that Pasteur started when he told us about germs and stoked the fear that led to an offensive approach, yet no one is looking to negotiate an end to it.

That's what I suggested in February of 2003 in my article "The next step in infectious disease: taming bacteria," published in *Medical Hypotheses*. Negotiating with microbes is done by blocking transmission. Blocking the transmission of social viruses is being done in countries like Poland that take steps to control fake news, but it is more often done by autocrats by just shutting down the opposition. We have the First Amendment rights that allow for both lies and truth, so it's up to us to determine what we follow. Understanding history, human behavior, and the Rotary's Four Way test are the best resources we have. They stop the transmission of errors that lead us down the path of virulence.

It's a paradigm for health that's simple and works exceptionally well for individuals as well as societies. It's built on the idea that defense is just as necessary as offense, and more, that taking a defense-first approach blocks transmission, whether it be a microbe or nuclear-armed nation, encouraging them to adapt in friendlier ways. For too long, we have fallen victim to the lizard-brain mentality of fighting that pervades atmospheres of threat and danger. We can do better.

A little education can go a long way, too, by exposing people to the methods used to manipulate them. The right environment for learning can quickly produce a generation of geniuses and innovators who may think of solutions we cannot even dream of now. That education can also immunize the next generations against the fear tactics and stresses that benefit defectors. It can strengthen defenses and build resistance against the opportunistic infections of Social Darwinism and neoliberalism.

We have the data that tells us what works and what does not. We have innovators who are using 21st-century thinking to solve our problems. And we have the threat of a long decline in national strength and even the threat of societal collapse to motivate us to do better. Talk with people on both sides of the political divide and you hear the same concerns. They want what we all want and have wanted since the beginning: life, liberty, and the pursuit of happiness. It is written right in the Preamble, and it's a promise we can keep because now we can control, we can understand, and we can have meaning. We can have coherence. We *can* do better.

Despite how things appear, my prognosis is optimistic for the health of ourselves and our society. Not only can we solve our problems and achieve our potential, but there is also something in our spirit aiding us from behind the scenes. It aided me in developing a revolutionary spray that optimizes nasal defenses. And my healthier patients showed me the value of fixing the cracks in our society.

As the voice of wisdom told me early one morning as I exited my dreams: "It's all the same." God created nature with its interrelated wholeness. We have now the principles of evolution, so we know how to play with it—and we are learning how to do so safely. All living and adapting systems need both offense and defense, warp and woof, and when one comes at the expense of the other, our balance is off. Imbalance leads to illness and fissures in society. As with health care in general, restoring the balance restores health. In our case, restoring the strength of our defenses, both physiologically for us and socially for our nation, is the way to restore our health.

We can, and we should, *make America healthy again.*

Endnotes

1 See for example, Ervin Laszlo & David Lorimer, *The Great Upshift: Humanity's Coming Advance Toward Peace and Harmony on the Planet.* Light on Light Press, Ft. Lauderdale, FL, 2023.

2 www.opensecrets.org/federal-lobbying

3 Knowles MR, Boucher RC. "Mucus clearance as a primary innate defense mechanism for mammalian airways." J Clin Invest. 2002 Mar;109(5):571-7. doi: 10.1172/JCI15217. PMID: 11877463; PMCID: PMC150901. See also: Wardzala CL, Wood AM, Belnap DM, Kramer JR. Mucins Inhibit Coronavirus Infection in a Glycan-Dependent Manner. ACS Cent Sci. 2022 Mar 23;8(3):351-360. doi: 10.1021/acscentsci.1c01369. Epub 2022 Feb 14. PMID: 35345395; PMCID: PMC8864775.

4 Reis, Gilmar, et al. "Effect of early treatment with ivermectin among patients with Covid-19." *New England Journal of Medicine* 386.18 (2022): 1721-1731.

5 H. Holden Thorp. "Generative approach to research integrity". *Science,* 11 August 2023, 381(6658)587.

6 www.nybooks.com/articles/2023/12/21/how-america-ends-and-begins-again-sherrilyn-ifill/

7 Brian Hare and Vanessa Woods. *Survival of the Friendliest: Understanding our Origins and Discovering our Common Humanity,* 2021. Random House Trade Paperbacks, New York.

8 Jeffrey Toobin. Circuit Breakers. New York Review of Books, March 7, 2024. P.16-18.

9 Christopher F. Karpowitz and Chad Raphael, *Deliberation, Democracy, and Civic Forums: Improving Equality and Publicity* (Cambridge: Cambridge University Press, 2016).

10 Homeostasis is the term that describes the body's ability to maintain an internal balance. It's why we have 'normals' for our temperature and all of the lab tests we run to make sure everything is working all right. Those seeing the value of different 'normals' when challenged by infection or other problems argue for "heterostasis"—different 'normals' for different conditions.

11 Ruxin JN. Magic bullet: the history of oral rehydration therapy. Med Hist. 1994 Oct;38(4):363-97. doi: 10.1017/s0025727300036905. PMID: 7808099; PMCID: PMC1036912.

12 Boss, J. "The medical philosophy of Francis Bacon (1561-1626)." *Medical hypotheses* vol. 4,3 (1978): 208-20. doi:10.1016/0306-9877(78)90003-8

13 Vanessa L. Bryant & Philip D. Hodgkin. "Life, death, and antibodies." Science, 13 Oct. 2017. 358 (6360):171-2. This is a review of an article in the same issue by C. T. Mayer, A. Gazumyan et al. "The microanatomic segregation of selection by apoptosis in the germinal center." Available at http://dx.doi.org/10.1126/science.aao2602

14 www.nih.gov/news-events/nih-research-matters/ancient-viral-dna-may-help-humans-fight-infections.

15 Glycans are a family of sugars and sugar complexes that coat our cells. They play a powerful role in immunity and infection.

16 Personal communication with Phillipe Hujole.

17 William Easterly, "Trust the Development Experts—All 7 Billion." The Brookings Institution, 2008.

18 Rowan Jacobsen. "Minds Everywhere." *Scientific American,* February 2024; **330**(2):44-51.

19 Molly Moore. "Top Israeli Officer Says Tactics are Backfiring." *Washington Post Foreign Service.* (October 31, 2003). Page A01.

20 Sara J Baker. *Fighting for Life,* 1940. Robert Hale Ltd. London. P. 157.

21 Todd Rose. *Collective Illusions: Conformity, Complicity and the Science of Why We Make Bad Decisions*, 2022. Hachette Books; New York.

22 Michael Fuoco, "What's in a President's Signature? Pittsburgh Expert Says, 'A Lot!'" *Pittsburgh Post-Gazette*, February 19, 2018.

23 Vivek Murtha. Our Epidemic of Loneliness and Isolation: The US Surgeon General's Advisory on the Healing Effects of Social Connection and Community.

24 Costerton, J.W., Geesey, G.G. and Cheng, K.J. (1978) How Bacteria Stick. Scientific American, 238, 86-95.

25 EL Bruger and CM Waters. "Bacterial Quorum Sensing Stabilizes Cooperation by Optimizing Growth Strategies". *Applied Environmental Microbiology;* 27 Oct. 2016. 82(22):6498-6506.Do

26 Ammons, Mary Cloud B et al. "Combined treatment of Pseudomonas aeruginosa biofilm with lactoferrin and xylitol inhibits the ability of bacteria to respond to damage resulting from lactoferrin iron chelation." *International journal of antimicrobial agents* vol. 37,4 (2011): 316-23. doi:10.1016/j.ijantimicag.2010.12.019

27 Bijay K. Khajanchi, Michelle L. Kirtley, Sheri M. Brackman, et al. "Immunomodulatory and Protective Roles of Quorum-Sensing Signaling Molecules N-Acyl Homoserine Lactones during Infection of Mice with *Aeromonas hydrophila*." *Infection and Immunity,* Jul 2011; 79 (7):2646-2657.

28 Graeber & Wengrow. Op. cit.

29 Ibn Khaldun. *The Muqaddimah: An Introduction to History,* trans. by Franz Rosenthal, edited and abridged by N. J. Dawood (Princeton, NJ: Princeton University Press, 1967.)

30 Jacques Monod, *Chance and Necessity: An Essay on the Natural Philosophy of Biology.* (New York: Knopf, 1974) p. ix.

31 Jacques Hadamard. *The Psychology of Invention in the Mathematical Field,* 1954. New York, Dover.

32 Anthony Tucker. "Max Perutz". The Guardian, Obituaries, February 7, 2002.

33 H. Holden Thorp. "Generative approach to research integrity". *Science,* 11 August 2023, **381**(6658)587. At other places in this book different types of organizational cultures are discussed: bureaucratic; pathological; and generative. The book hopes to build a generative culture, but the others seem to dominate our institutions where self-interest and self-protection dominate.

34 The American Academy of Arts and Sciences. *Our Common Purpose.* 2020.

35 Mark Bergen, "YouTube Executives Ignored Warnings, Letting Toxic Videos Run Rampant," *Bloomberg News*, April 2, 2019, https://www.bloomberg.com/news/features/2019-04-02/youtube-executives-ignored-warnings-letting-toxic-videos-run-rampant, accessed April 5, 2019.

36 There is a very good video demonstration of our airway defenses on YouTube; it's a video-microscopy of the mucociliary clearance process done by Fisher & Paykel, a New Zealand firm making humidifiers for sleep apnea devices. You can actually watch what happens when the humidity is reduced! It has been moved around so searching "mucociliary" and "Paykel" is the best way to find it.

37 Ezra Klein show, 31 May 2024.

38 Lev Vygotsky. *Thought and Language* (*Myshlenie y rech'*). Translated and edited by Alex Koulan. (Boston: MIT Press, 1986).

39 Benjamin Whorf, Language, Thought, and Reality. (Boston: MIT Press, 1956).

40 James Prescott is responsible for this bit on intimacy. In his work with monkeys he showed how a baby monkey learns trust by being carried and moving with another, attachment by being touched in a caring way—as in grooming—and intimacy by another's smell. Prescott worked at the NIH's Child Development section and came up with some very controversial ideas about the origins of violence that got him ostracized from the government. There is an online collection of his works at the German site: violence.de.

41 Julian Jaynes. The Origin of Consciousness in the Breakdown of the Bicameral Mind. (New York: Houghton Mifflin, 1990).

42 Hannah Arendt. *The Origins of Totalitarianism.* (New York: Houghton Mifflin Harcourt, 1951). P.473.

43 Chang-Yu Chang et al. Emergent coexistence in multispecies microbial communities. *Science,* 21 July 2023; 381(6655), 343-348. . DOI:10.1126/science.adg0727

44 Isabel Wilkerson. *Caste: The Origin of our Discontents,* 2020 (New York; Random House). See especially Chapter 8 The Nazis and the Acceleration of Caste.

45 U.S. elections face more threats from foreign actors and artificial intelligence. NPR. May 15, 2024. https://www,npr.org/2024/5/15/1251684195/election-interference-russia-china-senate-aritifical-intelligence

46 RD Sege, BS Siegel, AAP Council on Child Abuse and Neglect, and AAP Committee on Psychosocial Aspects of Child and Family Health. "Effective Discipline to Raise Healthy Children." *Pediatrics*, June 2018. 142(6): e201831 12.

47 Martin A. Nowak, "Five Rules for the Evolution of Cooperation." *Science;* 8 Dec 2006, 314(5805):1560-63. Nowak continues to explain the pressures to cooperate in more complex math.

48 Brian Hare & Vanessa Woods. "Survival of the Friendliest." *Scientific American*, February 2020; 323, (2): 58-63.

49 Cass Sunstein, "The Triumph of the Friendly: A Review of Brian Hare and Vanessa Woods, *Survival of the Friendliest*," *Journal of Bioeconomics* 22 (2020): 131–35.

50 Jonathan H. Turner, Alexandra Maryanski, Anders Klostergaard Petersen, and Armin W. Geertz. *The Emergence and Evolution of Religion: By Means of Natural Selection.* (New York: Routledge, 2018.) p.2

51 Resmaa Menakem, *My Grandmother's Hands* (Central Recovery Press, Las Vegas, NV. 2017). This book is an innovative disruptive approach to race relations.

52 P. J. Zhu, S. Khatiwada, Y. Cui, et al., "Activation of ISR Mediates the Behavioral and Neurophysiological Abnormalities of Down's Syndrome," *Science* 366, no. 6467 (November 13, 2019): 843–49.

53 B. Zhao, T. Li, Z. Fan et.al. Heart-brain connections: Phenotypic and genetic insights from magnetic resonance images. *Science* 380, no.6648 (2 June 2023): 934. Doi: 10.1126/science. abn6598.

54 Jimena Baleriola, Chandler A. Walker, Ying Y. Jean, et al., "Axonally Synthesized ATF4 Transmits a Neurodegenerative Signal across Brain Regions," *Cell* 158, no. 5 (August 28, 2014): 1159–72, https://www.sciencedirect.com/science/article/pii/S0092 867414008770.

55 Kressin NR, Glickman ME, Peterson ED, Whittle J, Orner MB, Petersen LA. Functional status outcomes among white and African-American cardiac patients in an equal access system. Am Heart J. 2007 Mar;153(3):418-25. doi: 10.1016/j.ahj.2006.11.019. PMID: 17307422.

56 Daniel Kahneman, *Thinking Fast and Slow* (New York: Farrar, Straus, and Giroux, 2011).

57 Jonathan Haidt, *The Righteous Mind: Why Good People Are Divided by Politics and Religion* (New York: Vintage, 2012).

58 Linda Liebender, Natascha Joubert, and Marie-Lynne Foucault, *Understanding Core Resilience*, Public Health Agency of Canada, November 2017, http://lindaliebenberg.com/wp-content/uploads/2017/11/PHAC-Resilience-Report-Final-Version-November-2017.pdf, accessed December 29, 2018.

59 H. I. McCubbin and J. M. Patterson, "The Family Stress Process: The Double ABCX Model of Adjustment and Adaptation," in *Social Stress and the Family: Advances in Family Stress Theory and Research*, ed. H. I. McCubbin, M. Sussman, and J. M. Patterson (New York: Haworth, 1983), 7–38.

60 Aaron Antonovsky, *Health, Stress, and Coping,* (Jossey-Bass Social and Behavioral Science Series, 1979). See also his *Unraveling the Mystery of Health: How People Manage Stress and Stay Well,* in the same series in 1987.

61 Emily Esfahani Smith, The Power of Meaning: Crafting a Life that Matters (New York: Broadway

62 Emily Underwood. "Lessons in Resilience." Science, 2 March 2018; **359**(6379): 976-9.

63 Elinor Ostrom. Governing the Commons: The Evolution of Institutions for Collective Action. (Cambridge: Cambridge University Press. 1990).

64 Available at: americanindian.si.edu/environment/pdf/01_02_Thanksgiving_Address.pdf

65 Sarah Fader, "What Is the Learned Helplessness Psychology Definition?" Better Help, www.betterhelp.com/advice/behavior/what-is-the-learned-helplessness-psychology-definition/, accessed August 5, 2019.

66 Martin E. P. Seligman, Christopher Peterson, and Steven F. Maier, *Learned Helplessness: A Theory for the Age of Personal Control* (New York: Oxford University Press, 1995).

67 Personal communication with a son who served in both Bosnia and Afghanistan and was involved with these training programs as an NCO.

68 John Lewis, "Together, You Can Redeem the Soul of Our Nation." *New York Times*, July 30, 2020.

69 Ruby K. Payne, *A Framework for Understanding Poverty* (Highlands, TX: aha! Process, 1996).

70 Rema Hanna. "Technology beats corruption: Biometric smart cards help reduce corruption in cash transfer programs in India." *Science,* 20 January 2017, **355**(6322):244-5.

71 Joseph Stiglitz. *There is no Invisible Hand.* The Guardian, Dec. 20, 2002.

72 Edward Chancellor, "Waiting to Deflate," *The New York Review of Books*, Sep. 9, 2021. Pp 50-53.

73 Ivan Tyrrell. "The Uses and Abuses of Hypnosis." The Human Givens Institute. Published online at https://www.hgi.org.uk/resorces/delve-our-extensive-library/ethics/uses-and-buses-hypnosis.

74 Hari Sridhar, Guy Beauchamp, Kartik Shanker: *Why do birds participate in mixed species foraging flocks? A large-scale synthesis.* Animal Behaviour, Volume 78, Issue 2, 2009, Pages 337-347

75 John Roberts, *2019 Year-End Report on the Federal Judiciary*, https://www.supremecourt.gov/publicinfo/year-end/2019year-endreport.pdf, accessed February 5, 2020.

76 Gordon Allport. The Nature of Prejudice, 1954 (Cambridge, MA; Addison-Wesley).

77 Chiara Cordelli, "Justice as Fairness and Relational Resources," *The Journal of Political Philosophy* 23, no. 1 (2015): 97.

78 Cordelli's reference is to James Moody, "Race, School Integration, and Friendship Segregation in America," *American Journal of Sociology* 107 (2001): 679–716.

79 Derek Black, "Leaving White Nationalism," *Southern Poverty Law Center Intelligence Report*, August 21, 2013, https://www.splcenter.org/fighting-hate/intelligence-report/2013/leaving-white-nationalism, accessed November 30, 2019.

80 George Wallace, Martin Luther King Jr., and the power of forgiveness. Commentary. *Christian Science Monitor,* 14 January 2021.

81 Orentlicher, David, "Judicial Consensus: Why the Supreme Court Should Decide Its Cases Unanimously" (2022). Connecticut Law Review. 523. https://opencommons.uconn.edu/law_review/523

82 Haidt, op. cit., 105.

83 Peter T. Coleman. "The U. S. is Suffering from Toxic Polarization. That's Arguably a Good Thing." Scientific American, April 2, 2021.

84 Tali Mendelberg, Christopher F. Karpowitz, and J. Baxter Oliphant, "Gender Inequality in Deliberation: Unpacking the Black Box of Interaction," *Perspectives on Politics* 13, no. 1 (2014): 1–27.

85 Turner, Maryanski et al. op.cit. P. 2.

86 H. Holden Thorpe. "Generative approach to research integrity." *Science,*11 Aug. 2023; 381(6658)587. See note 5 for my description of a bureaucratic culture.

87 Jared Bernstein, "Savings Incentives for the Poor," *The American Prospect*, April 16, 2003, https://prospect.org/article/savings-incentives-poor, accessed September 2, 2019.

88 Linda Gorman, "The History of Health Care Costs and Health Insurance," Wisconsin Policy Research Institute 19, no 10 (October 2006), http://www.wpri.org/BI-Files/Special-Reports/Reports-Documents/Vol19no10.pdf, accessed October 13, 2008.

89 Robert D. Putnam, Bowling Alone: The Collapse and Revival of American Community (New York: Simon & Schuster, 2000).

90 Christopher H. Achen and Larry M. Bartels, *Democracy for Realists: Why Elections Do Not Produce Responsive Government* (Princeton, NJ: Princeton University Press, 2017).

91 Ibid., 298.

92 Eric C. Ellis. "New views on ancient peoples." A review of David Graeber and David Wengrow. The Dawn of Everything: A New History of Humanity, Farrar, Straus, and Giroux, 2021, in science 26 November 2021; 374 (6571):1061.

Index

Made in United States
Orlando, FL
10 November 2026

90498873R00134